CONTEMPORARY ISSUES IN COLORECTAL SURGICAL PRACTICE

Edited by **Yik-Hong Ho**

Contemporary Issues in Colorectal Surgical Practice
Edited by Yik-Hong Ho

Published by InTech

Janeza Trdine 9, 51000 Rijeka, Croatia

Publishing Process Manager Dragana Manestar

Technical Editor Teodora Smiljanic

Cover Designer InTech Design Team

Additional hard copies can be obtained from orders@intechopen.com

Contemporary Issues in Colorectal Surgical Practice, Edited by Yik-Hong Ho
p. cm.
ISBN 978-953-51-0257-1

Meet the editor

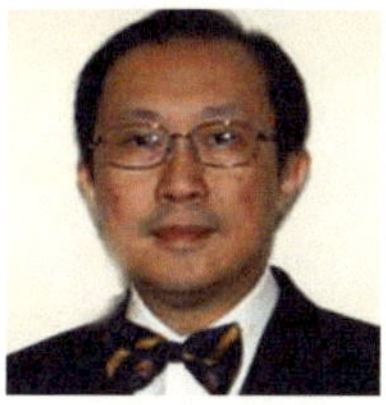

He is actively involved in colorectal surgical training as well as in academic supervision of postgraduate research doctorate degrees. His contributions to the medical literature include over 180 peer reviewed primary publications and 26 textbook chapters. He is associate editor for International Surgery and chairman of the editorial board for Techniques in Coloproctology, Yik-Hong is a member of several medical societies and is presently the World Corporate Secretary of the International College of Surgeons.

Contents

Preface

The practice of colorectal surgery is a rapidly evolving discipline which continually seeks to evaluate and incorporate new emerging technological advances and management concepts into routine day to day practice. This is necessary to achieve continued excellence in service delivery, particularly for patients with complex problems. When these techniques and concepts eventually withstand the robust testing of wide-spread routine surgical practice, they become assimilated into traditional textbooks. Nonetheless, there is a time lag because traditional textbooks require substantial time in production and readership distribution which is something that the on-line electronic medium overcomes, particularly when the latter is focused on selected key topics.

In recent years, significant progress in colorectal surgery has been made which includes laparoscopic techniques, pre-operative management, emergency colorectal surgery, fast track multimodal recovery, management of complex wound problems and colorectal cancer follow-up. "Contemporary Issues in Colorectal Surgical Practice" aims to bridge the gap between the journal article and the traditional textbook in these areas.

Dr. Yik-Hong Ho
Professor & Head of Surgery, School of Medicine & Dentistry,
James Cook University, Townsville,
Australia

Part 1

Perioperative Management

1

Preoperative Preparation in Colorectal Surgery

Arne-Christian Mohn
Haugesund Hospital, Helse Fonna HF
Norway

1. Introduction

In august 1954 Robert J. Gosling Read said at the 59th Annual Convention of the National Medical Association, Washington, D.C: "...Through the personal knowledge of the patient's life history and interest he (*the good family physician*) has offered advice based on common sense rather than specialized training. This is the concept of accelerated recovery..."

This was the first time in the literature the concept was used. Interesting enough, several points of today's enhanced recovery are also common sense since all items are not evidence based. Evidence-based medicine is defined as the integration of best research evidence with clinical expertise and patient values to optimise clinical outcomes and quality of life.[1]

The concept returned in surgery in 1990. Krohn et al[2] published from Good Samaritan Hospital in Los Angeles a four days discharge from hospital after open-heart surgery. He called it rapid sustained recovery. This was the first paper on enhanced recovery after surgery (ERAS).

In 1994 Hartford Hospital and Baystate Medical Center[3] introduced the term "fast-track surgery" which included 1: preoperative education, 2: early extubation, 3: methyl-prednisolon sodium succinate before surgery followed by dexamethasone for 24 hours postoperatively, 4: prophylactic digitalization, metoclopramide HCL, docusate sodium, and ranitidine HAL, 5: accelerated rehabilitation, 6: early discharge, 7: a dedicated fast-track coordinator to perform both daily telephone contact and a 1-week postoperative examination and 8: a routine 1-month postoperative visit with a PA or MD. This showed a systematically control of all patients and a multimodal focus to enhance the recovery time. But all the interventions were not evidence based and the study was an observational study.

Why didn't the literature focus on recovery before1990?

One reason was that until the 1980´s the preoperative preparation was optimizing the organ function medically to tolerate the narcosis, bowel preparation to avoid anastigmatic leakage and infection and disinfection of the surgeons' hands and the patients' skin. There were no systematic antibiotics given, no thrombi-prophylaxis and no epidural anaesthetics.

Another reason was the lack of methodical trials and evidence based medicine on ancillary procedures. Variations in surgical procedures and peri-operative care have been recognised since the early 1980s and are generally interpreted as evidence of uncertainty among practitioners regarding optimal care.[4] How different surgeons or hospitals provided the procedures varied enormously, leading to and "expertise bias". They tended to be accepted with little question and which, fore some surgeons, had become indispensible rituals. Most of the surgery was done the way you learned it from your mentor. He had his own meaning based on his experience and a standard saying was: "In our hospital we do it my way" or said by Edmund Burke: "custom reconciles us to everything."

Further, randomised trials to peri-operative care questions were often difficult or impractical to perform. A valid randomised controlled trial may also be impossible in many circumstances and may limit the generalisability of the results.

In the 1990s there was a change. The main reason was the specialization. Earlier the surgeon did the anaesthetics themselves, but today we have specialists in this area, which make us treat patients. The securing of a safe anaesthesia during operations is more important than ever before, partly because of the mere number of operations, and partly because of the greater extent to which other operative risks – haemorrhage, shock and infection – have been overcome. The risk from the anaesthetic is now so very small that the joint aim of the surgeon and anaesthetist to abolish it altogether is not far from being accomplished.[5] The specialty of anaesthesia has seen major advances thanks to the development of safer anaesthetic agents, improved knowledge of pain physiology and pain management, and incorporation of a better understanding of peri-operative patho-physiology into peri-operative care. Concomitantly, development of minimally invasive surgery has further reduced stress responses and pain, thereby providing potential for enhanced recovery. However, an increasing proportion of elderly patients with organ dysfunction have led to demands for further reductions in postoperative complications and the costs of treating them.

The transition from inpatient surgery to ambulatory procedures has proceeded at a rate that was unthinkable a few decades ago, but could all surgical procedures ultimately be done on an outpatient basis?[6] The forthcoming years will, as before, pose several challenges for anaesthetists to improve peri-operative care and to take part in the multidisciplinary collaboration of fast-track surgery. Anaesthetists should consider the development of "peri-operative medicine" as a multidisciplinary effort that should not involve conflict between the anaesthetic and surgical specialities, but rather serve as a mutual platform for improvement of peri-operative care. All together there are more and more emphasis on the joint aim: peri-operative preparations and recovery.

Through the 1980´s and the 1990´s, evidence based medicine became the state of the art, but still it is troublesome to change the way of thinking.

2. ERAS

Kehlet et al gave some answers to these questions in 1997[7]: He focused on the improvements on the administration of opioid analgesics in new ways, such as continuous or on demand intravenous or epidural infusion. These methods allowed lower total opioid dosages, provided a more stable concentration of opioid and correspondingly better analgesic effects, and also fewer unwanted side effects. The introduction of rapid short acting volatile anaesthetics, opioids, and muscle relaxants also facilitated expansion of ambulatory surgery for minor to moderate procedures. The emphasis on ambulatory surgery and accelerated surgical stay programs, both with a focus on early recovery of organ function and provision of functional analgesia, provided an opportunity for a reappraisal of opioid use in these settings. However, the same techniques may be used to facilitate early recovery and decreased need for prolonged monitoring and stay in recovery and high dependency wards after major procedures.

The key factors that keep a patient in hospital after uncomplicated abdominal surgery include the need of parenteral analgesia (persisting pain), intravenous fluid (persisting gut function), and bed rest (persisting lack of mobility).[8] ERAS change the way of thinking to minimal these factors.

Traditionally the complication rate in colorectal surgery is between 20-40%. The hospital stay is between one and two weeks.[9,10] Early clinical pathways had showed reduced length of stay in major surgery.[11] Kehlet published his first results[8,12,13] with a hospital stay of two days after colonic surgery. He established the concept accelerated recovery and started to compile an interest group, which later became the ERAS-group. Studies showed reduction in hospital stay, reducing ileus and cardiopulmonary complications.[10,13-23] Also in rectal cancer surgery the peri-operative "fast-track" multimodal rehabilitation program is effective and safe.[24,25] Randomised controlled trials (RCT) have showed the same results,[19,20,22,23,27-29] though Behrns patients were discharged on liquid diets.

Advances in peri-operative patho-physiology have indicated multi-factorial reasons for post-operative morbidity[30], length of stay and patient recovery. It is therefore required to deal with these causes by multifaceted interventions. First of all, the patient's medication must be optimized according to organ function like cardiac disease, chronic obstructive lung disease, diabetes mellitus etc. Further the patient must be evaluated according to malnutrition. Malnutrition can prolong the stress response and increase the likelihood of complications. Likewise, heavy drinkers and smokers should abstain from alcohol and smoking a month before surgery if possible. Otherwise they have higher incidence of complications. Thereafter the treatment should focus on pain relief, reducing stress response and reducing nausea and vomiting. Further on the patients should avoid hypothermia, immobilization and semi-starvation. Finally, the postoperative ileus should be minimized. There are reasons to believe that including as many ERAS elements as possible in a clinical pathway may result in a cumulative effect and contribute to enhanced recovery in patients.[31]

The major premise behind fast-track surgery is that patients regain function more rapidly and that this allows a reduction in the period during which the patient is unable to perform activities of daily living.[21]

Better adherence to the elements of the ERAS protocol is crucial to improve surgical outcome. Nearly all, preoperative and per-operative ERAS interventions, influenced postoperative outcomes beneficially.[32] Patients with high adherence to the ERAS protocol had a 25% lower risk of postoperative complications and nearly 50% lower risk of postoperative symptoms delaying discharge. They also had a higher tendency toward reaching length of stay within the target limits compared with patients operated on under less optimal ERAS protocol adherence. As the enhanced recovery field develops, certain interventions may turn out to be nonessential. However, before omitting specific components in the protocol, such a decision should be based on a closer understanding of the importance of each element in the program.

Many of the peri-operative interventions that have been widely adopted into clinical practice are supported by very limited evidence. For a number of interventions the data are either limited in quantity or quality, or are inconsistent. Systematic reviews should be

Elements	**Guidelines**
Preoperative information	Oral and written information to patients and relatives. Achieve patient management. Patient education before and after surgery.
Bowel preparation	No bowel preparation is necessary before colon surgery. Preparation still before rectal surgery.
Admission	The day before or operation day. Oral supplements given at home before admission.
Preoperative fasting	Fasting only 2 hours before surgery, food and milk rinks 6 hours before.
Carbohydrate loading	Drinks the evening before (800ml) and 2-3 hours before surgery (400ml)
Preoperative medication	Paracetamol (1g x 4) reduces postoperative pain, Alvimopan (12mg x2) reduces postoperative ileus
Preoperative anticoagulation	No-risk - no anticoagulation. Moderate-risk once a day at least 5 days. High-risk once a day 28 days
Preoperative antibiotics	Oral and intravenous or intravenous only. Cephalosporins (2g) or combination doxycycline (0,4g) and metronidazol (1,5g).
Preoperative epidural anaesthesia	Mid-thoracic EDA* during surgery (bolus and continous infusion) and EDA or PCA$ postoperatively for 2-3 days reduces PONV#, ileus, pain, and hospital stay.
PONV	Peroperative and early postoperative oxygen. On moderate-risk TIVA% or an antiemetic drug. In high-risk combination og TIVA and dexamethasone.
Surgical incisions	Less is better, laparoscopy even best.
Nasogastric tubes	Have no place routinely in elective colorectal surgery
Peroperative normothermia	Normothermia during surgery, reduces wound infections
Postoperative fluid management	Restricted, goal-directed fluid therapy is preferably
Drainage of the abdominal acity	No need in colon surgery. In rectal surgery still needed.
Urinary drainage	1 day after colon surgery and about 3 days after low-rectal surgery
Postoperative ileus	Complex aetiology with many contributors, but opioids exacerbate the ileus
Postoperative nutritional care	Oral intake 4 hours after surgery and normal food intake the day after.
Mobilization	Out of bed operation day and 6 hours the day after and thereafter

*EDA = epidural anaesthesia, $PCA = patient-controlled anaesthesia, #PONV = postoperative nausea and vomiting, %TIVA = total intravenous aenesthesia

Table 1. **Elements of ERAS (Enhanced Recovery After Surgery)**

conducted with the same methodological rigour expected for randomised controlled trials. Systematic reviews conducted under the auspices of Cochrane Collaboration have an established methodology and peer review process, and they may be less prone to bias than non-Cochrane systematic reviews.[1]

There is supportive evidence from studies that enhanced recovery programs should be considered as standard peri-operative care.[33] Still, there are controversies. Meta-analysis,[31,34,35] show reduction of complications, but not major complications. There may be a decrease, but it is not statistical significant. One reason may be the lack of robust RCT's. The reduction of hospital stay is real and the readmission rate does not increase. However, a Bayesian meta-analysis showed significant reduction in hospital stay, complications and no difference in readmission rates and mortality.[36] A Bayesian model has a number of advantages like full allowance for all parameter uncertainty, the ability to include other pertinent information that would otherwise be excluded, and the ability to extend the models to accommodate more complex, but frequent occurring, scenarios.[37]

The debate is still going and the conclusion is unclear, but ERAS should be considered the new standard. The markedly shortened hospital stay in fast-track rehabilitation should change the capacity of operative departments considerably. At the same time denotes the implementation of fast-track rehabilitation a paradigm shift away from invasive postoperative monitoring and regulation attempts of today's intensive care medicine to intensified pain therapy and reinforced physical rehabilitation.

Today the ERAS-group has consensus guidelines. They recommend as many elements as possible (for instance 17 out of 20), but as mentioned above – still several elements are highly debatable. We will therefore in this chapter discuss the elements mentioned in Table 1, to see if there are evidence today to change the way of preparing the patients and go into the next area: Optimize the preparation, peri-operative treatment, the logistics and the recovery.

But first, we will look at the concepts stress response and insulin resistance.

3. Stress response and insulin resistance

Surgical stress response is a major contributing factor to postoperative morbidity. Advances in surgical technique and peri-operative management the last years have allowed better control of the stress response intra-operatively and improved patient outcome.

Surgical stress response is mediated via neuro-endocrine mechanisms leading to alterations in protein homeostasis (increased catabolism), hyper-metabolism, altered carbohydrate metabolism (increased gluconeogenesis and insulin resistance) and increased lipolysis.[20]

The underlying hypothesis is that the reaction to a physical stress depends in part on the metabolic state at the onset of the stress. In many of its features, postoperative insulin resistance resembles type 2-diabetes mellitus. The reduction in insulin sensitivity develops after surgery in patients with and without type 2 diabetes.[38]

A state of insulin resistance has been confirmed in several different types of stress, including burn injury, accident trauma, and sepsis. During the 1990s studies of insulin resistance in elective surgery have been performed.[39] The degree of postoperative insulin resistance was significantly correlated with the length of stay postoperatively. The duration of surgery was closely associated to the relative decrease in whole body insulin sensitivity. These findings suggest that the relative change in insulin sensitivity is related to the degree of surgical stress.[40]

4. Preoperative information

It is very important to inform both the patient and relatives days before the surgery. An effective implementation and a consequent huge rate of compliance are essential in terms of achieving uniformity of patient management. A thorough information orally and a written preadmission information describing what will happen during their hospital stay, what they have to expect, and what their role in their recovery, are essential.[8,41] The success relies on the patients understanding and appreciating their responsibilities.[42] Preoperative education may reduce anxiety and aid in coping, generally enhancing postoperative recovery with an earlier return of gastrointestinal motility after surgery.[43,44] Some patients require extensive education in issues relating to stoma care, self-monitoring for signs of dehydration, and sexual function. This education starts before operation and continues after the operation.[45]

It is well established that intensive preoperative patient information can facilitate postoperative recovery and pain relief, particularly in patients who exhibit most denial and the highest level of anxiety.[9] Teaching the patient to cope with pain and the importance of pain control and the expectation of some degree of nausea are important task to understand before surgery. Patients should also understand the importance of getting out of bed the evening of the operation or the envisioned discharge on the third or fourth postoperative day.

Further on an evaluation of the home environment is important beforehand. In that way it is easier to plan an early, realistic discharge day. Family or caregiver support is crucial to ensure a safe transition from hospital to home and to decrease the risk of readmission.

A cornerstone in the achievement is motivated surgeons, anaesthesiologists and study nurses.[9,46] Fast-track surgery requires a multidisciplinary, concentrated and coordinated effort, with nurses as essential to the success of these programs.[47,48] The dedicated and motivated team consists of anaesthesiologists, surgeons, residents, dieticians, physiotherapists, social workers, dieticians, and nursing team. The nurses should concentrate on individual tasks and spend much time on managing complications as they occur. They must challenge the traditional nursing practices and expend this role to avoid that patients become passive recipients of care. The nurses partner with the patient to achieve well-defined goals to improve patient's outcome.

Changes also need to be made to organisational strategies and the medical professionals involved in pre, intra and especially postoperative care require support, perhaps via continuing education.[47] A protocol is not enough and the importance of this collaboration has been widely described.[5,9,11,13,19,46,49-51]

- Orally and written information to reduce anxiety and postoperative pain
- Achieve patient management and avoid passive recipients of care

5. Bowel preparation

It was unquestionably a great convenience to the surgeon to operate on an empty bowel rather than on one loaded with faeces. It was also supposed through a century that operations on the bowel, especially those involving a suture line or an anatomises, were safer and less likely to be associated with gross contamination and sepsis if the intestine is in a relatively or completely empty condition.[52] The assumption, which formed the basis for the practice of mechanical bowel preparation prior to major colorectal surgery, was so widely accepted as sensible and logical, that nobody saw the need of any really stringent scrutiny. Until recently it was thought that vigorous preoperative mechanical cleansing of the bowel (mechanical bowel preparation), together with the use of oral antibiotics, reduced the risk of septic complications after non-emergency (elective) colorectal operations. Mechanical bowel preparation was performed routinely prior to colorectal surgery until 1972, when this procedure started to be questioned. Even though ES Hughes in 1972[53] concluded in a randomised clinical study that vigorous mechanical preparation was not necessary, most surgeons continued the bowel cleansing until late 1980s.

But in the late 1980s some started to question the necessity of bowel cleansing when using intravenous antibiotics.[54] The cleansing was time consuming and associated with discomfort. Even though Burke[55] stated that bowel preparation does not influence outcome after elective colorectal surgery and a review concluded with limited evidence in the literature to support the use of mechanical bowel preparation[56], still until late 1990s it was standard along with antibiotics preoperatively. The question wasn't answered until two well-designed randomized clinical trials were performed and printed in The Lancet and Br J Surg in 2007.[57,58]

Reviews and meta-analysis cannot show higher leakage rate with than without bowel preparation. Some studies and even meta-analysis have shown the opposite with higher frequencies after preparation,[59,60] but the evidence based answer today is that there are no differences and therefore it is not necessary with any preparations before colon surgery.[61] It is too early to conclude on rectal surgery, so still one may do the preparation before the surgery here. Further research on mechanical bowel preparation or enemas versus no preparation in patients submitted for elective rectal surgery and laparoscopic colorectal surgery is warranted.

There are also some controversies about what kind of preparation to use. No bowel preparation method meets the ideal criteria for bowel cleansing prior to surgery. The new generation of bowel purgatives include oral sodium phosphate preparations and polyethylene glycol-electrolyte lavage solutions. Both are well tolerated by the patients with the oral sodium phosphate preparation as the most preferred because of less fluid to drink for the patients and possibly more effective,[62,63] but there are still some safety issues without a clear solution. Both cleansing methods make some electrolyte disturbances even though it seems like the polyethylene glycol-electrolyte lavage solutions are less dangerous.[64] Therefore adequate hydration is important before, during, and after bowel preparation.[65]

Furthermore, in children and elderly, patients with kidney disease or decreased intravascular volume, and those using medicines that affect renal perfusion or function (diuretics, angiotensin converting enzyme (ACE) inhibitors, angiotensin receptor blockers (ARBs), and possibly non-steroidal anti-inflammatory drugs (NSAIDs)) should not use oral sodium phosphate. There is a possibility to develop acute phosphate nephropathy. They should instead use polyethylene glycol-electrolyte lavage solutions.[66]

- No need for bowel preparation in colon surgery
- Still need in rectal surgery

6. Admission

Earlier the patients admitted to the hospital two days before surgery. On the admission day they were given a full liquid diet, and on the day before surgery, a clear liquid diet. Bowel cleansing was given the day before.

Today the history of the patient and co-morbidity are evaluated in an outpatient manner by the surgeon and the anaesthetist. The oral carbohydrate feeding and/or protein feeding are done home by the patient. It is a common view that nutritional support in the peri-operative phase is associated with decreased morbidity, particularly in severely nutritionally depleted patients.[9,67] Patients receiving oral nutritional supplements over an extended peri-operative period lost significantly less weight than those who received no supplements or postoperative supplements only. The incidence of minor complications was significantly lower than in those receiving no supplements or preoperative supplements only. The benefit of outcome occurred independently of nutritional status.[68]

The use of laxatives is still debatable, as the standard measure of return of bowel function would be the ability to tolerate oral feeding rather than just bowel movement.[31]

The patient, at home, may handle the injection of anti-coagulant, the evening before surgery. If the patient lives distant from the hospital, he can be admitted the day before surgery or stay at a hospital hotel.

- Admission the day before or operation day
- Patients receive and administrate oral nutrition supplements at home

7. Preoperative fasting and carbohydrate loading

The overnight fasting routine was first suggested in 1848 after Hannah Greener's death in Winlaton, as a result of the first reported death following general anesthesia.[69] Later the same century it was suggested that a better preparation for the patient was to allow a cup of tea or beef tea some hours before the operation.[70] In the early 1900s, reports of complications from aspirations resulted in the strict recommendation of nil by mouth.[66] General anaesthetic reduces reflexes that stop regurgitated gastric juices reaching the lungs. As this can be dangerous, people were often advised to have nothing to eat or drink from the midnight before surgery.

The main reason for questioning the nil by mouth rules was to improve patient's well being, by reducing thirst and for caffeine drinkers avoiding headaches from withdrawal symptoms. Norway was the first country to adopt new guidelines in 1993, the Norwegian Consensus Guidelines for preoperative fasting in elective surgery, and a national survey was performed three years later, which showed no increase in aspirations due to the new routines.[72] Fasting before general anaesthesia aims to reduce the volume and acidity of stomach contents during surgery, thus reducing the risk of regurgitation-/aspiration.[73] Recent guidelines have recommended a shift in fasting policy from the standard 'nil by mouth from midnight' approach to more relaxed policies, which permit a period of restricted fluid intake up to 2 hours before surgery. Food or drinks containing milk make the emptying slower and need six hours.[74,75] Emptying of the stomach usually occurs within less than 90 minutes in elective patients after consumption of clear fluids, and after a 12,5% carbohydrate loaded drink 120 minutes.[76]

Practice has been slow to change. There was no evidence to suggest a shortened fluid fast results in an increased risk of aspiration, regurgitation or related morbidity compared with the standard 'nil by mouth from midnight' fasting policy. Permitting patients to drink water preoperatively resulted in significantly lower gastric volumes. Clinicians should be encouraged to appraise this evidence for themselves and when necessary adjust any remaining standard fasting policies (nil-by-mouth from midnight) for patients that are not considered 'at-risk' during anaesthesia. Some people are considered more likely to regurgitate under anaesthetic, including those who are pregnant, elderly, and obese or have stomach disorders. More research is needed to determine whether these people can also safely drink up to a few hours before surgery.[75]

Beverages including water, tea, coffee, or juices without fruit meat cannot be expected to cause any major changes in metabolism, and thus, even with the new and more liberal fasting guidelines, the patient will be operated in a metabolic state of fasting. Infusions of carbohydrates before elective abdominal surgery were shown to improve postoperative insulin sensitivity.[77] Carbohydrate feeding given shortly before elective colorectal surgery displayed less reduced insulin sensitivity (reduced insulin resistance) after surgery compared to patients who were operated after an overnight fast[40] and not associated with aspiration.[78]

The patients were given 800 ml 12,5% carbohydrate drink (malto-dextrin) the evening before the operation and another 400 ml about 2-3 hours before the operation. Insulin resistance has been shown to be an independent factor explaining the variation in length of stay.[79] This study showed that preparation with a carbohydrate-rich drink increased preoperative wellbeing compared with intake of placebo (water) or overnight fasting. These drinks lead to reduced anxiety and significantly reduced postoperative hospital stay, and a trend towards earlier return of gut function when compared with fasting or supplementary water.[8,32,38,80] This earlier return of bowel function may be a contributory factor for shorter hospital stay. Consumption of an appropriate potion composed of water, minerals and carbohydrates offers some protection against surgical trauma in terms of metabolic status, cardiac function and psychosomatic status.

- No fluid intake 2 hours before surgery, milk drinks and food until 6 hours before
- Carbohydrate drinks (>12,5%) the evening before and 2-3 hours before surgery

8. Preoperative medication

Patients should not receive pre-anaesthetic anxiolytic or analgesic medication.[8] Paracetamol used, as preoperative medication to reduce postoperative pain is well established. The use of diclofenac to strengthen the effect (postoperatively) has caused unwanted side effects both in animal studies and retrospective clinical studies.[81] This study showed significant more anastomotic leakages. Therefore it is recommended to use other non-steroid anti-inflammatory drugs or opioid antagonists like Alvimopan.

Alvimopan is a novel, oral, peripherally acting antagonist, a μ-opioid receptor that has limited ability to cross the blood-brain barrier and is currently being evaluated for the management of postoperative ileus.[82] The use is 12 mg 2 hours before surgery and then twice daily beginning on first postoperative day until hospital discharge or for a maximum of 7 days of postoperative treatment. Alvimopan act within the gastrointestinal tract and does not affect the centrally mediated analgesia. Alvimopan significantly accelerate gastrointestinal recovery in bowel resection patients; reduce postoperative morbidity rates, hospital stay, and rates of hospital readmission[83] with a mean daily opioid consumption of 26 mg. However, opioids provide better pain control compared with other analgesics such as anti-inflammatory drugs.

Glucocorticoids (GCs) are well known for their analgesic, anti-inflammatory, immune-modulating, and antiemetic effects, although the mechanisms by which glucocorticoids exert their action are far from clarified.[84] Preoperative GCs decrease complications—including infectious complications specifically and length of stay after major abdominal surgery. Although inflammation is a necessary precursor for healing, it is the excessive amplitude of the inflammatory response after major abdominal surgery that is thought to contribute to postoperative morbidity and delay recovery. GCs do not seem to increase the risk of complications in colorectal surgery.[85] As an intervention; administration of GCs is inexpensive and simple allowing for clinical implementation without difficulty. Earlier there was not found a significant effect or no effect on postoperative nausea and vomiting and pain in studies. In the concept of enhanced recovery, the effects have been found[84] but Fukami et al found no effect in a randomized controlled trial[86] Another trial found that 8 mg dexamethasone preoperatively has no significant effect on reducing postoperative inflammatory response and also does not improve outcomes of colorectal surgery.[87]

The analgesic effects of GCs are provided through inhibition of the phospholipase enzyme and accordingly blockage of both the cyclooxygenase and the lipoxygenase pathway in the inflammatory chain reaction. The mechanism by which GCs alleviate nausea and vomiting is not fully understood, but the effects are probably centrally mediated via inhibition of prostaglandin synthesis or inhibition of the release of endogenous opioids.

Postoperative fatigue appears to be an important problem following only certain forms of surgery. Preoperative administration of dexamethasone resulted in a significant reduction in early postoperative fatigue, associated with an attenuated early peritoneal cytokine response. Peritoneal production of cytokines may therefore be important in postoperative recovery.[88] The reduction in fatigue was moderate and was associated with a diminished peritoneal pro-inflammatory cytokine reaction on day 1, supporting the hypothesis that peritoneal inflammation is an important contributor to fatigue after major abdominal surgery.

Because of divergence in the trials, we need larger randomised trials before we can recommend the use of GCs before surgery.

- Paracetamol given preoperatively reduce postoperative pain
- Alvimopan is an alternative to reduce postoperative ileus

9. Preoperative anticoagulation

Venous thrombo-embolism (VTE) is the most common preventable cause of death in surgical patients. Thrombo-prophylaxis, using mechanical methods to promote venous outflow from the legs and antithrombotic drugs, provides the most effective means of reducing morbidity and mortality in these patients. Despite the evidence supporting thrombo-prophylaxis, it remains underused. The reasons for its underuse are not fully understood, but those having abdominal surgery are often considered to be at a lower risk than orthopaedic patients. In addition, there are still concerns about an increased risk of bleeding complications.[89,90]

The overall incidence of venous trombo-embolism (VTE) without anticoagulation is 20-25% for patients more than 40 years old in general surgery. For patients having cancer, the incidence slightly rise to 30-40%.[89-93] Fatal embolism occurred in about 1%. After low molecular weight heparin (LMWH) the incidence of VTE is 6% and fatal embolism 0,01%.[92,94,95] Complication rates are low and should not prevent the use of prophylaxis in most patients.[91] Patients undergoing surgery of the large bowel and the rectum have a considerable risk of developing vascular complications expressed as venous thrombosis and/or thrombosis in the lungs (pulmonary embolism). These complications can lead to lifelong impaired venous function in the legs or occasionally sudden postoperative death. The clinical importance of asymptomatic proximal and distal deep vein thrombosis (DVT) remains uncertain and controversial. Unrecognised DVT may lead to long-term morbidity from post-phlebitic syndrome and predispose patients to recurrent VTE. Because VTE in hospitalized patients often is asymptomatic, it is inappropriate to rely on early diagnosis. Furthermore, non-invasive tests, such as compression ultrasonography, have limited sensitivity for a diagnosis of asymptomatic DVT. The high mortality rate in patients with asymptomatic proximal DVT underscores its clinical relevance and supports asymptomatic proximal DVT as an appropriate endpoint in clinical trials.[96,97] Thrombo-prophylaxis is, therefore, the most effective strategy to reduce morbidity and mortality from VTE in surgical patients. Low-dose unfractioned heparin (UFH) and LMWH appear to be equally effective and safe in this patient group, and either agent can be used. Because patients with underlying cancer are at higher risk, it is reasonable for them to use elastic stockings in conjunction with these agents.

The advantage of LMWH is that it can be administered once daily and it is less likely to cause heparin-induced thrombocytopenia and thrombosis than standard heparin preparations. Among the most important risk factors are a previous history of thrombotic disease, advanced age (risk levels increase above 40 years), prolonged immobility, and coexisting cancer and its treatment.[90]

In low-risk patients, who undergoing minor or relatively short operations, are less than 40 years old and with no additional risk factors, no prophylaxis is necessary except early and frequent mobilization.

In moderate-risk patients who are more than 40 years old and undergoing major surgery with no additional risk factors, LMWH given once daily (>3,400 anti-Xa Units) or graduated compression stockings used properly, is sufficient for at least 5 days.[98]

In high-risk patients more than 40 years old with additional risk factors, LMWH given once daily supplied with graduated compression stockings may be sufficient. But the length of anticoagulation has been discussed. A review demonstrates that this combined treatment also is effective within the high-risk group of patients undergoing surgery of the large bowel or rectum.[97]

In addition to ensuring optimal timing for the initiation of prophylaxis, it is also important to establish the duration of prophylaxis. A review suggests that prophylaxis should be administered for at least one month after surgery.[99] The ENOXACAN II study showed, at least in high-risk patients, a significant benefit of an extended 4-week prophylactic period compared with the standard 1-week regimen, with no increase in adverse effects, confirmed by a meta-analysis.[87,100,101] It is now some evidence that late thrombotic events can occur up to 6-7 weeks after operation.[90] Even if there are no difference in mortality, the patients with lower limb DVTs have almost 60% higher relative risk of suffering from post-thrombotic syndrome. Furthermore there are associations between higher 90 days mortality and asymptomatic proximal DVT, which explain the large number of fatal pulmonary emboli in autopsy series.

In laparoscopic surgery and fast-track surgery there are not any RCTs to tell if it is sufficient to give the prophylaxis for a shorter period. Until then one must carefully include selected high-risk patients, major cancer surgery or they who have previously had VTE, to continuing thrombo-prophylaxis after hospital discharge with LMWH for up to 28 days.

It should be emphasized that epidural analgesia per se reduces thrombo-embolic complications by 50% in lower body procedures, but this has not been demonstrated after abdominal procedures.[8]

- In low-risk patients no prophylaxis is necessary
- In moderate-risk patients LMWH once daily or compression stockings, 5 days
- In high-risk patients LMWH supplied with stockings recommended for up to 28 days

10. Preoperative antibiotics

Without any prophylactic antibiotics, one may consider more than 40% wound infections after colorectal surgery, or at least 27% found by Raahave et al[102] with extensive bowel cleansing. In that case it is unethical to operate without any coverage as pointed out in the first meta-analysis on the field.[103] The conclusions were that the chosen antibiotics were not the crucial point, but the timing, coverage and duration were the most important variables. The latest Cochrane Analysis confirms this.[104]

The antibiotics must cover the copious mixture of both anaerobic and aerobic species, which are in the large intestinum. [104] The optimal drug should be one that is not used as a first-line choice in the treatment of surgical infection. But the most common drug used worldwide is cephalosporin, which also is used in the treatment of infections. However, doxycycline, used in Scandinavians studies[105,106] and still used in Scandinavia, is not an antibiotic commonly used in the treatment of established surgical infection, nor is it prominently associated with causing C. difficile colitis, and it is not expensive. But to cover the anaerobic agents, doxycycline is given together with metronidazol with the same limitations as cephalosporin. Doxycycline has not been studied extensively in comparison to other established gold-standard antibiotic recommendations, but perhaps it should be. According to timing it is well accepted that one hour before surgery is optimal and there is no need for a second dosage because of increased risk of resistant organisms and Clostridium difficile colitis. A combination of oral and intravenous antibiotics seemed to be better than intravenous only, but because of current recommendations before surgery; it should probably be given intravenously.

- Antibiotics given intravenously or a combination of oral and intravenous antibiotics
- Cephalosporin (2g) or Doxycycline (400mg) and Metronidazol (1,5g) preoperatively

11. Preoperative Epidural Anaesthesia (EDA)

Prevention and treatment of postoperative pain is the central goal of interdisciplinary anaesthetists and surgeons. The use of epidural anaesthesia is not for pain control only. Effective analgesia reduces the intensity of autonomous and somatic reflexes, but of importance is the blockade of afferent fibres from the surgical site in order to positively modulate posttraumatic stress reaction either by peripheral nerve blockade, spinal or epidural analgesia.[41] It leads to a modification of the endocrine metabolic action after major surgical procedures, whilst postoperative inflammation is not affected. Mid-thoracic epidural activated before the onset of surgery also blocks stress hormone release and attenuates postoperative insulin resistance.[8]

Both afferent pain fibres and sympathetic efferent fibres contribute to ileus. Because postoperative pain activates the autonomic system and indirectly causes adverse effects on various organ systems, blockage of these pain signals both intra-operatively and postoperatively with epidural anaesthesia and analgesia can blunt the stress response and minimize the effect of surgery on bowel motility.[107,108] There is experimental evidence that the sympathectomy produced by local anaesthetics is associated with increased gastrointestinal blood flow. Shortened duration of postoperative ileus after abdominal operations using these techniques may be translated into decreased length of stay and patient satisfaction.[109]

Regional anaesthesia and analgesia, particularly neural blockade, produce a host of benefits for surgical patients, accelerates recovery of organ function including gastrointestinal and pulmonary function, decreased cardiovascular demands, superior pain relief, reduce the amount of general anaesthetic used (allowing faster recovery), and allows intensified early mobilisation.[49,107,110] Administration of epidural local anaesthetics to patients undergoing laparotomy reduces gastrointestinal paralysis compared with systemic or epidural opioids, with comparable postoperative pain relief. Addition of opioid to epidural local anaesthetic may provide superior postoperative analgesia with activity compared with epidural local anaesthetics alone, and can be accomplished with less toxicity than either class of drug.[1,109-111] The activation of nociceptive afferent and sympathetic efferent nerves are believed to reduce pain and peri-operative opioid requirements, which may lead to reduced postoperative nausea and vomiting (PONV).

Most important may be the significant and prolonged response in the stress response when the epidural anaesthesia is continued postoperatively. To produce the benefit reliably, it appears that epidural analgesia with local anaesthetics should be instituted before the surgical stress and continued until postoperative ileus has resolved, typically 2-3 days later. This peri-operative analgesia may contribute to lower risk of death after surgery. The low risk of serious adverse consequences suggest that many high-risk patients undergoing major intra-abdominal surgery will receive substantial benefit from combined general and epidural anaesthesia intra-operatively with continuing postoperatively epidural analgesia.[112,113] The effect of additional epidural opioid on gastrointestinal function is so far unsettled even if it is indicated that epidural local aesthetic/opioid provide the most superior treatment.[8,110]

The effect of using epidurals on the postoperative pain outcome was investigated in two studies using visual analogue score (VAS).[19,20] Improved postoperative pain relief is important for patient comfort and may decrease the hospital stay and lead to reduction in morbidity. Improved blood flow consequent on sympatholysis has additional potential benefits, including a reduction in thrombo-embolic complications.[1]

Some studies have shown that thoracic epidural analgesia with a mixture of local anaesthetics and opioids, in contrast with patient-controlled anaesthesia (PCA) IV opioids, provides superior pain relief and contributes to a faster restoration of bowel function.[49,108] However, other trials with patients on a fast-track care pathway with intravenous PCA analgesia did not get further benefits with use of a pre-emptive thoracic epidural.[111,114] In a Cochrane Database analysis,[110] although epidural administration of local anaesthetics was found to accelerate gastrointestinal recovery and reduce nausea after abdominal surgery compared with epidural or systemic opioids, it did not reduce length of stay compared with patient-controlled opioid analgesia.[83]

And therefore, research continues to find the optimum infusion (constituents, concentration and total volume) and the optimum timing and duration of infusion to find significant difference between mid-thoracic epidural analgesia peri-operatively and PCA on the length of stay, too.

A practical problem may evolve during operations. The blockade of these fibres leads to hypotension and the laparotomy intensifies low blood pressure. Then it is very tempting to fill up with intravenous fluid to achieve normal tension. But, as we will discuss later, the risk is intravenous fluid overload. Therefore remember, peroperative hypotension is safely treated with vasopressors.

- Mid-thoracic EDA during surgery and EDA or PCA postoperatively at least for 2-3 days, reduces PONV, postoperative ileus and pain and therefore reduces hospital stay
- Addition of opioid to epidural local anaesthetic provide superior analgesia

12. Preventing and treating postoperative nausea and vomiting

Postoperative nausea and vomiting and postoperative ileus are well-recognized syndromes that lead to significant morbidity and prolong hospitalization. Anaesthesia is given worldwide to more than 75 million surgical patients annually. Untreated, one third of surgical patients suffer from PONV.[115] Patients often rate PONV as worse than postoperative pain. Volatile anaesthetics, nitrous oxide and opioids appear to be the most important causes. Female gender, non-smoking and a history of motion sickness and PONV are the most important patient specific risk factors.[116] Vomiting increases the risk of aspiration and has been associated with suture dehiscence, oesophageal rupture, subcutaneous emphysema, and bilateral pneumothorax. Numerous patho-physiological mechanisms are known to cause nausea or vomiting but their role for postoperative nausea and vomiting is not quite clear.

Intra-operative and early postoperative supplemental oxygen may reduce nausea and vomiting after colonic surgery, and the effect may be as affective as odansetron.[5]

The use of short-acting volatile and intravenous anaesthetics can influence the postoperative course favourably and reduces the incidence of PONV markedly. At a moderate risk the use of total intravenous anaesthesia (TIVA) or an antiemetic is reasonable because PONV frequently delays discharge from post-anaesthesia care units. In very high-risk patients one may justify the combination of several prophylactic antiemetic interventions. The necessary doses are usually a quarter of those needed for treatment.[116] Management techniques such as TIVA cannot be used once PONV is established. A reasonable treatment strategy in high risk patients would be to use dexamethasone and total intravenous anaesthesia as first- and second-line prophylaxis for postoperative nausea and vomiting, leaving serotonin antagonists as a rescue treatment.[115] But dexamethasone, prevents PONV only when given in the beginning of surgery, probably due to reducing of surgery-induced inflammation. "Rescue" treatment, like serotonin antagonists, is ineffective when the same drug has already been used as prophylaxis. Prophylaxis may therefore be preferable to treatment of established PONV.

- Oxygen supplement intra-operative and early postoperative reduces PONV
- Moderate-risk patients may respond to TIVA or an antiemetic drug peroperative
- In high-risk patients a combination of TIVA and dexamethasone peroperative

13. Surgical incisions

To minimize the inflammatory process and pain, the incisions should be reduced to a minimum. Transverse incisions may cause less postoperative pain and better pulmonary function.[117] Therefore laparoscopic incisions may be even better.[118,119] Laparoscopic colon resections have showed advantages over conventional surgery. Blood loss is less; pain, treated with epidural or patient-controlled on demand analgesia, is less intense; time to return of bowel function is less, lung function is improved with reduced postoperative stay in hospital and improved quality of life in the first 30 days. The operation time is still longer with laparoscopic surgery than with conventional surgery. Re-operation is not more likely after laparoscopic surgery and general complications in the lungs, heart, urinary tract or deep vein thrombosis (DVT) were similar with the two surgery techniques. Wound infections were less in laparoscopic patients.[120-123]

Despite the minimally invasive nature of laparoscopy, host physiologic responses to stress are still variably activated. The sane gamut of metabolic, hormonal, inflammatory, and immune responses activated by open surgery are also induced by laparoscopy, but to a lesser degree and proportionate to the extent of surgical injury.[124]

- Small incisions give smaller inflammatory responses. Laparoscopy even better.

14. Nasogastric intubation

In 1933 Wangensteen and Paine[125] wrote: "It is now twenty-four years since Westermann first used the duodenal tube in the relief of postoperative distension of peritonitis. With the introduction of the smooth tipped duodenal tube for nasal intubation by Levin in 1921 and satisfactory demonstration of the source of gas in postoperative dissention by McIver and his associates in 1926 as being largely swallowed air, the relief of postoperative distension through employment of the duodenal tube has become a matter of general practice." Thereafter the nasogastric tube was used routinely.

The practice was based largely on tradition and perception that nasogastric decompression protected patients from postoperative complications such as nausea, vomiting, aspiration, wound complications, anastomotic leak, and therefore allowed an earlier hospital discharge. Formerly, some used nasogastric tubes for 24 hours when using or more. Many of the early studies advocated nasogastric decompression allowing the patients ad libitum oral intake with the nasograstric tube in place, a practice that would not be advocated by most surgeons today.[126]

Routine nasogastric decompression was widely practiced after elective laparotomy. But the use of nasogastric tubes affect patients considerably. Studies have shown that nasogastric tube decompression does not shorten the duration of ileus and may, in some cases, contribute to postoperative complications such as nasal and pharyngeal injury, fever, atelectasis, increased gastric reflux, regurgitation, and pulmonary infections.[82,127] RCTs could not show any relevant benefit. Although patients may develop abdominal distension or vomiting without nasogastric tube, this is not associated with an increase in complications or length of stay.[126]

The beginning of modifications in practice came after a RCT by Olesen et al 1984,[128] which showed earlier passage of flatus without using tubes and no differences were found regarding duration of postoperative ileus, severity of postoperative paralysis, as measured by occurrence and duration of nausea and vomiting, postoperative per oral fluid intake, and time for defecation. And a meta-analysis showed that patients not having routine tube use had an earlier return of bowel function, a decrease in pulmonary complications and an insignificant trend toward increase in risk of wound infection. On the other hand routine use may decrease the risk of wound infection and subsequent ventral hernia.[127] Although abdominal distension and vomiting are increased without nasogastric decompression, nasogastric tube insertion is required in only 5% to 7% of selectively treated patients,[129] whereas nasogastric tube replacement postoperatively is required in 2% of routinely treated patients. Routine use of nasogastric decompression after elective operations is today not supported by the literature.[127]

- Nasogastric tubes have no place routinely in elective surgery today

15. Preventing intra-operative hypothermia

When compared with normothermic controls, the degree of mild hypothermia has been associated with a twofold to threefold increase in surgical wound infections.[5]

Maintenance of normothermia is critical for the surgical patient. Hypothermia has been shown to impair coagulation and increase the stress response and cardiovascular demands. Using forced-air warmer devices and providing adequate clothing and covering during surgery, can help to reduce postoperative wound infections, blood loss, untoward cardiac and overall rate of nitrogen excretion and catabolism.

- Maintenance of normothermia reduces wound infections

16. Peri-operative fluid management

Intravenous fluid and electrolytes are given to resuscitate the patient from losses sustained during surgery and to maintain homeostasis during periods when oral intake may not be possible. In major surgery, the need for intravenous fluid is greater. However, the optimum fluid replacement strategy remains controversial.

Avoidance of intravenous fluid overloading is an important element in many protocols. Current practice in fluid regimens has been based on 40-year old concepts.[130] It was postulated a decrease in functional extracellular fluid after surgery but this decrease has never been found.[27,131]

However, a study on dogs back in 1937, showed that a modest positive salt and water balance caused weight gain after elective colonic surgery and was associated with delayed recovery and gastrointestinal motility, increased complication rate and hospital stay.[132] The same was found in humans in 2002.[133] An excess of salt and water may lead to more complications than restriction of fluid.

Francis Moore first recommended restriction in fluid regimen.[134] He argued that the metabolic-endocrine response to trauma, (conservation of salt and water), required a fluid restriction. Shires' recommendations have led to 4-6 litres or more intravenous substitution during surgery and 24 hours after, despite minimal blood loss. In contrast, "dry" regimen has been considered beneficial in thoracic surgery.[135] Intravenous fluid overload or excess early sodium and fluid prescription during and after surgery have been shown to give adverse outcome like decrease in muscular oxygen tension and delayed recovery of gastrointestinal function after segmental colonic resection with moderate fluid restriction. Postoperative weight gains after intra-operative fluid overload have been associated with poor survival and complication.[27,136,137] The pattern peri-operative intravenous fluid administration has a major effect upon cardio-respiratory and anastomotic complications, and restricted peri-operative intravenous fluid management and a preoperative carbohydrate drink were found to be of specific importance for beneficial outcomes.[32]

Factors that allow successful use of restricted intra-operative fluid regimen include preventing the patient from coming to the theatre in a dehydrated state by avoiding bowel preparation or excessive duration of preoperative fasting. There was no apparent difference between the effects of fluid-restricted and standard or liberal fluid regimens on outcome in patients undergoing elective open abdominal surgery in a meta-analysis. However, patients managed in a state of fluid balance fared better than those managed in a state of fluid imbalance.[50,138] It is clear that restriction of intravenous fluid during and after operation is safe in well-hydrated patients undergoing major elective abdominal surgery[50] without finding any significant effect on postoperative gastrointestinal function or hospital stay between conservative intra-operative fluid control, and postoperative restriction of fluids and sodium. On the other hand, restricted postoperative IV fluid management, as performed in one trial, in patients undergoing major abdominal surgery, appears harmful as it is accompanied by an increased risk of major postoperative complications and a prolonged postoperative hospital stay.[139] But this study was not an ERAS protocol and had no multimodal approximation.

Some studies have used Doppler-guided fluid administration as goal-directed therapy. Oesophageal Doppler-guided fluid management may improve outcome following major intra-abdominal surgery. However, comparison with fluid restriction strategies, including a cost-effectiveness analysis is required.[139] Evidence regarding use of Doppler-guided fluid administration is limited by heterogeneity in trial design, and recent advances in surgical techniques and peri-operative care may largely offset the initial clinical benefits observed.[140]

All together when using standardized definitions, restricted rather than standard fluid amount according to current textbook opinion, and goal-directed fluid therapy rather than fluid therapy guided by conventional hemodynamic variables, reduce morbidity after colorectal resection.[141]

- Avoiding unnecessary bowel preparation or excessive duration of preoperative fasting
- Restricted, goal-directed fluid therapy seems to be the best regimen

17. Drainage of peritoneal cavity following colonic anastomosis

Drainage of chest empyema and ascites go back to the Hippocratic era. Ambroise Pare was the first to describe drainage of the abdominal cavity, but abdominal drainage had probably been used in practice earlier.[142] During the last 2 centuries, surgeons also used drains for prophylactic purposes. Prophylactic drains have been employed to remove intra-peritoneal collections such as ascites, blood, bile, chyle, and pancreatic or intestinal juice.[143] Another assumed potential function of prophylactic drains is their signal function to detect early complications, such as postoperative haemorrhage and leakage of enteric suture lines.

F. Manley Sims[144] was the first surgeon who used prophylactic drains after gynaecological operations in the end of 19th century. Since that time, surgeons have routinely used prophylactic drainage of the peritoneal cavity after abdominal surgery.[143] Many surgeons use prophylactic drainage after colorectal anastomoses worldwide to prevent anastomotic dehiscence by evacuating fluid collections. Previous authors have suggested that drainage is important to prevent accumulation of exudative fluid, but randomised trials that examined pelvic fluid accumulation in the presence and absence of a drain demonstrated no reduction in fluid accumulation despite the presence of a functioning drain.[145,146] And there is no evidence that fluid exuded from the pre-sacral fascia will remain in the pelvis rather than communicate with the free peritoneal cavity, and may therefore not be susceptible to capture by a pelvic drain. In addition, a drain will usually not serve to control an anastomotic leak as many surgeons expect. The fact is that only in very few instances leaks among drained patients in evaluated studies, pus or faeces emerging from the drain.[146,147]

These traditional practices can impede mobility and cause discomfort and thereof increased morbidity. The use should be selective and not used routinely. Many surgeons continue to place a prophylactic drain in the pelvis after completion of a colorectal anastomosis, despite considerable evidence that this practice may not be useful. If drainage tubes first have been inserted they are normally left in situ for several days until drainage ceases. During the last 3 decades, surgeons have made effort to investigate the value of prophylactic drainage after abdominal surgery in controlled randomised clinical trials. Despite evidence-based data questioning prophylactic drainage in many instances, most surgeons around the world continue to use them on a routine bases. A possible reason for the persistence of practice may be that the surgeons are not convinced by the negative results of the existing trials. The relatively small sample size and the rarity of the outcomes in these studies limit their power to exclude a true benefit, should one exist.[142]

The large variability of drainage duration may indicate the need for future RCT focused on drainage duration, especially on short-term drainage (24-48 hours). But reviews and meta-analysis of the literature found no evidence that justifies routine drainage of colon and rectal anastomosis after uncomplicated surgery today.[143,147] They showed no difference in all outcome measures (mortality, clinical anastomotic dehiscence, radiological anastomotic dehiscence, wound infection, reoperation, length of hospital stay, extra-abdominal complications).[145,148]

However, due to the lack of statistical power after stratification to the level of the anastomosis, anastomosis in the pelvic still may need short-time drainage. Especially concerning the increase in the rate of neoadjuvant radiotherapy and the increase of Gy used, the reactive hyperaemia should indicate the need of drainage.

- No drainage after colon surgery is needed
- Because of increasing use of radiation, drainage may be used in pelvic surgery

18. Urinary drainage

Some prefer to leave the catheter in situ for several days after surgery, until the patient is fully mobilized. Others remove it the day after surgery on colonic resections, leaving the catheter for seven days after pelvic surgery. Few RCTs are available to define the optimal duration of such drainage, but patients require a shorter period of urinary catheterisation, are able to mobilise more quickly, and had an earlier return of gut function in optimized pathways.[5,20] One study recommend in major low-rectal operations, urinary bladder drainage to be limited to about 3 days and to 1 day after types of colonic surgery.[5]

- 1 day after colonic surgery, about 3 days after low-rectal operation

19. Prevention of postoperative ileus

The aetiology of postoperative ileus is complex, and major intrinsic contributing factors include surgical stress (i.e., from physical manipulation of the bowel), secretion of inflammatory mediators and endogenous opioids in the gastrointestinal tract, and changes in hormone levels and electrolyte and fluid balance, pharmacological agents such as inhalation anaesthetics, and use of opioids for postoperative analgesia implying that both stimulation of nociceptive afferent and sympathetic efferent nerve pathway initiate ileus.[82,108,113] Opioids are the most widely prescribed analgesics used to treat postoperative pain. However, opioids bind to μ-opioid receptors within the gut, exacerbating postoperative ileus.[83] The μ-opioid receptors have been the subject of investigative targets to block and thereby add a pharmacologic adjunct that has previously been lacking.[149]

Postoperative ileus is defined as a disruption of the normal peristaltic motion of the gut, resulting in failure to propel intestinal content through the gastrointestinal tract. Symptoms associated with postoperative ileus include abdominal distension and bloating, nausea and/or vomiting, lack of bowel sounds, gas and fluid accumulation in the bowel, delayed passage of flatus and stool, and inability to tolerate solid diet. Small bowel ileus resolves within hours of manipulation, but gastric and colonic motor function does not return until 48 to 72 hours postoperatively.[23] It is due to inhibition of extrinsic motility regulation in the colon. The potential benefits from prompt resolution of postoperative ileus may include reduction in the incidence of bowel complications, the potential for more rapid return to normal bowel function, improved patient comfort, reduced length of stay, and reduced healthcare costs.[82]

Postoperative ileus has been shown reduced in fast-track groups[47] even though Lewis[67] found an increased risk of vomiting among patients fed early. This meta-analysis did not include patients in an ERAS protocol. And again, including many ERAS elements in a clinical pathway may result in a cumulative effect not found studying one at the time.

The greatest advance in limiting postoperative ileus to date has probably resulted from the expanded use of laparoscopic surgery and the advantage of limiting tissue trauma. Animal and clinical trials have demonstrated significant reductions in postoperative ileus after laparoscopic colectomy compared with open techniques, which translate into decreased hospital stay.[149]

Postoperative ileus is one of the most common causes of prolonged length of hospital stay. Furthermore, postoperative ileus may be a significant contributing factor for hospital readmission.

- Opioids exacerbating postoperative ileus, but the aetiology is very complex and many elements may contribute

20. Postoperative nutritional care

Standard before ERAS was no oral alimentation until flatus passed, and then progressive diet was initiated. Initially, clear fluids were given, followed by full liquids, and than a regular diet. On average, fluids were commenced on the third or fourth day, with discharge of the patient on the seventh or the eighth day following surgery. Intravenous fluid was administered until the patient was able to drink ad libitum. Until intestinal activity was demonstrated to have reasserted itself in a normal way, by the detection of vigorous peristaltic sounds on regular auscultation of the abdomen and the passage of flatus per rectum, normal diet was banned.

The immediate advantage of caloric intake could be a faster recovery with fewer complications. In the 1990s, early oral intake after elective abdominal colorectal surgery was found safe and was tolerated by the majority of the patients, though they were on a clear liquid diet on the first postoperative day, and advanced to a regular diet within the next 24-72 hours,[150,151] and there was a significant attenuation in gut mucosal permeability.[152] Early studies showed early feeding as a key factor in reducing acute hospital stay,[153,154] and later studies reduced infection rate and the length of stay, but did not significantly reduce mortality.[1] A recent meta-analyse by Lewis et al[155] concluded with reduced mortality, but increased vomiting. However, the trend was in the direction of reduced complication rate and hospital stay. There is no advantage keeping the patient "nil by mouth".

Reduction in complication rates may explain the shortened length of stay as might faster return of gastrointestinal function upon early commencement of enteral feeding.[78] Early enteral feeding is predicated on radiologic and electro-physiologic studies that indicate a return of small bowel function in 4 to 8 hours post incision, right colon function by 24 hours and left colon function by 72 hours. Severity in duration of the atony can be attenuated by laparoscopy, reduction in opioid-based anaesthesia and analgesia, as well as blockade of the sympathetic reflex circuit through effective continuous thoracic EDA with local anaesthetics.

Early oral intake has become a routine feature in management after elective colonic surgery. And when is it appropriate to start? Patients should be encouraged to commence oral fluid intake 4 hours after surgery.[8]

- There is no advantage keeping the patient "nil by mouth".
- Patients should be encouraged to commence oral fluid intake 4 hours after surgery and normal food intake the day after surgery

21. Early mobilization

Previously, active movements were encouraged in bed after surgery. On the second or the third evening, the patient was usually helped out of bed for a few minutes whilst the bed was made. Thereafter the ambulation was gradually increased.

However, immobilization, over a longer period, can lead to organ dysfunction, loss of lean body mass, reduced muscle power and fatigue.[20] Bed rest not only increases insulin resistance but also decreases pulmonary function and tissue oxygenation and give an increased risk of thromboembolism.[8] To avoid pulmonary complications caused by reduced pulmonary function due to immobilization and reduced tissue oxygenation, mobilizing the patients as soon as possible is important. Mobilization starts on the day of surgery or on the first operative day.[107]

Patients should be nursed in an environment that encourage independence and mobilization. A care plan that facilitates patients being out of bed for up to 2 hours on the day of surgery and 6 hours thereafter is recommended.

To be considered fit for discharge patients had to be apyrexial, fully mobile, passing flatus or faeces, and using oral analgesics only for pain control.[50]

- Out of bed the operation day and 6 hours first operation day and thereafter

22. Economic consideration

In colorectal surgery, cost-analysis of enhanced recovery protocols is limited. Two early clinical pathway programmes proved useful in standardising patient care and reducing costs,[11,48] and were probably instrumental in the development of modern ERAS protocols.[156] None of these studies addressed the set-up costs of an ERAS protocol nor provided a detailed breakdown of where cost savings were achieved in the postoperative recovery phase. However, there has been a huge paradigm shift in postoperative care principles in colorectal surgery since that time, making the cost-analysis reported in those studies inapplicable to current programmes.

Cost-effective analysis has shown that an ERAS programme is a very cost-effective intervention in elective colonic surgery in the setting of an elective hospital.[156] Another case-control study by King et al 2006[157] focussing on quality-of-life after colonic and rectal surgery, showed in hospital stay half as long as those receiving conventional care, with no increased morbidity, deterioration in quality of life or increased cost.

Evidence from the literature, supports the view that the ERAS pathway seems to reduce the overall healthcare cost.[114,158,159] The largest reduction was in expenses for nursing care, although significant reduction were recorded also in costs of laboratory tests, medications (pharmacy), medical service and other expenses.[114] From a health economics point of view, the data suggests that, with the decrease of complications and hospital stay and similar readmission rates, the cost of treatment per patient would be significant lower for those treated with an ERAS pathway than those receiving traditional care, despite the need for dedicated staff to implement the pathway.[33]

23. Implementation

Improved adherence to the standardized multimodal ERAS protocol is significantly associated with improved clinical outcomes following major colorectal cancer surgery, indicating a dose-response relationship.[32] In spite of a large evidence base for peri-operative care aiming to alleviate postoperative catabolism and organ dysfunction, surgical patients remain exposed to unnecessary starvation, suboptimal stress reduction, and fluid overload.[160]

Although the concept of multimodal postoperative rehabilitation seems rationale and simple, implementation in daily practice has been surprisingly slow so far. This can be partly explained by the need to break with longstanding traditions such as preoperative fasting, postoperative advancement of oral feeding and delayed mobilization.[47] Partly that the ERAS concept as such possibly appears elusive because the relative contribution of each intervention in the program remains uncertain. The most plausible explanation is that a successful multimodal rehabilitation program requires the reorganisation of peri-operative care, with increased collaboration between the patient, anaesthetist (acute pain service), surgical nurse and surgeon. Furthermore, major efforts must be made for educational programmes, with emphasis on peri-operative patho-physiology, as well as a revision of traditional postoperative care programmes with drains, gastrointestinal tubes, catheters, restrictions etc.[48]

The step from best evidence to best practice is simple. However, most of the time it is not, and we need various strategies targeting obstacles to change at different levels, which could even present conflicting values for individual practitioners. Therefore, changes in clinical practice are only partly within doctor's control. Obstacles to change are generally not only in the professional setting but also in the patient, the organisation of care processes, resources, leadership, or the political environment. The prevailing professional and organisational culture towards quality determines the outcome to a large extent.[161]

For instance, patients were not expecting to go home in less than seven days and surgeons were cautious with early discharge.[108] Patients made an early functional recovery, but discharge was generally 2 days later.[9] Strict discharge criteria were met approximately 1,5 days before actual discharge. Social factors, patient's needs, and physician care all influenced the actual discharge date or length of stay.[107]

Introducing ERAS protocols usually requires a major shift in clinical routines, and many units may have difficulties in making all these changes at once. The delay in integrating novel management strategies with routine practice may be ascribed to the time required to develop guidelines, the implementation process, the target group of professionals, the patients, the cultural and social setting, and the organizational and economic environment.[9] Much may be achieved simply by raising the quality of surgical care according to existing evidence. In many ways, this is far more difficult task than simply doing more research.[4]

Nevertheless, some of the elements in the ERAS program, such as omission of routine bowel preparation for colonic resections, no routine use of postoperative drains, early removal of nasogastric tubes, and early feeding and mobilization, have already been incorporated in traditional care. The effect of the different peri-operative ERAS interventions as well as the importance of adherence to the protocol in terms of clinical outcomes, such as postoperative symptoms, morbidity, and length of stay (LOS), remain unclear.[32]

If you would like to start tomorrow to change practice and implement evidence, prepare well: involve the relevant people; develop a proposal for change that is evidence based, feasible, and attractive; study the main difficulties in achieving the change, and select a set of strategies and measures at different levels linked to that problem; of course, within your budget and possibilities. Define indicators for measurement of success and monitor progress continuously or at regular intervals. And, finally, enjoy working on making patients' care more effective, efficient, safe, and friendly.[161]

24. References

[1] Meeran H, Grocott MPW: Clinical review: Evidence-based perioperative medicine? Critical Care 2005, 9:81-85

[2] Krohn BG, Kay JH, Mendez MA et al: Rapid sustained recovery after cardiac operations. J Thorac Cardiovasc Surg. 1990 Aug; 100(2):194-7.

[3] Engelman RM, Rousou JA, Flack JE 3rd et al: Fast-track recovery of the coronary bypass patient. Ann Thorac Surg. 1994; 58(6):1742-6.

[4] Urbach DR, Baxter NN: Reducing variation in surgical care. BMJ 2005; 330;1401-1402.

[5] Kehlet H, Wilmore DW: Multimodal strategies to improve surgical outcomes. Am J Surg 2002: 183: 630-41.

[6] Kehlet H & Dahl JH: Anaesthesia, surgery, and challenges in postoperative recovery. Lancet 2003; Vol 362: 1921-8.

[7] Kehlet H: Multimodal approach to control postoperative pathophysiology and rehabilitation. Br J Anaesth 1997; 78: 606-17.

[8] Fearon KC, Ljungqvist O, Von Meyenfeldt M et al: Enhanced recovery after surgery: A consensus review of clinical care for patients undergoing colonic resection. Clinical Nutrition 2005 24, 466–477

[9] Maessen J, Dejong CHC, Hausel J et al: A protocol is not enough to implement an enhanced recovery programme for colorectal resection. Br J Surg 2007; 94:224–31

[10] Nascimbeni R, Cadoni R, Di Fabio F et al: Hospitalization After Open Colectomy: Expectations and Practice in General Surgery Surg Today (2005) 35:371–376

[11] Archer SE, Burnett RJ, Flesch LV et al: Implementation of a clinical pathway decreases the length of stay and hospital charges for patients undergoing total colectomy and ileal pouch/anal anastomosis. Surgery 1997;122(4): 699.705.

[12] Bardram L, Funch-Jensen P, Jensen P et al: Recovery after laparoscopic colonic surgery with epidural analgesia, and early oral nutrition and mobilisation. Lancet 1995; Mar 25 (345): 763.

[13] Basse L, Jakobsen DH, Billesbølle P et al: A Clinical Pathway to Accelerate Recovery after Colonic Resection. Ann Surg 2000; 232(1):51–57

[14] Kiran RP, Delaney CP, Senagore AJ et al: Outcomes and prediction of hospital readmission after intestinal surgery. J Am Coll Surg. 2004 Jun;198(6):877-83.

[15] Kehlet H & Mogensen T: Hospital Stay of 2 days after open sigmoidectomy with a multimodal rehabilitation programme. Br J Surg 1999; 86: 227-30.

[16] Hensel M, Scwenk W, Bloch A et al: The role of anaesthesiology in fast track concepts in colonic surgery. Anaesthesist 2006; 55(1): 80-92.

[17] Basse L, Thorbøl JE, Løssl K et al: Colonic Surgery with Accelerated Rehabilitation or Conventional Care. Dis Colon Rectum 2004; 47: 271–278

[18] Jakobsen DH, Sonne E, Andreasen J, Kehlet H: Convalescence after colonic surgery with fast-track vs conventional care. Color Dis 2006; 8 (10), 683–687.

[19] Anderson ADG, McNaught CE, MacFie J et al: Randomized clinical trial of multimodal optimization and standard perioperative surgical care. Br J Surg 2003; 90: 1497–1504.

[20] Gatt M, Anderson ADG, Reddy BS et al: Randomized clinical trial of multimodal optimization of surgical care in patients undergoing major colonic resection. Br J Surg 2005; 92: 1354–62.

[21] Nygren J, Hausel J, Kehlet H et al: A comparison in five European Centres of case mix, clinical management and outcomes following either conventional or fast-track perioperative care in colorectal surgery Clin Nutr (2005) 24, 455–461

[22] Delaney CP, Zutshi M, Senagore AJ et al: Prospective, randomized, controlled trial between a pathway of controlled rehabilitation with early ambulation and diet and traditional postoperative care after laparotomy and intestinal resection. Dis Colon Rectum. 2003 Jul;46(7):851-9.

[23] Behrns KE, Kircher AP, Galanko JA, Brownstein MR, Koruda MJ. Prospective randomized trial of early initiation and hospital discharge on a liquid diet following elective intestinal surgery. J Gastrointest Surg 2000;4:217–21.

[24] Delaney CP, Fazio VW, Senagore AJ et al: “Fast track” postoperative management protocol for patients with high co-morbidity undergoing complex abdominal and pelvic colorectal surgery. Br J Surg 2001; 88: 1533-8.

[25] Schwenk W, Neudecker J, Raue W et al: "Fast-track" rehabilitation after rectal cancer resection Int J Colorectal Dis. 2006 Sep;21(6):547-53.

[26] Teeuwen PHE, Bleichrot RP, Strik C et al: Enhanced Recovery after Surgery (ERAS) Versus Conventional Postoperative Care in Colorectal Surgery. J Gastrointest Surg 2010; 14: 88-95.

[27] Khoo CK, Vickery CJ, Forsyth N et al: Aprospective Randomized Controlled Trial of Multimodal Perioperative Mangaement Protocol in Patients Undergoing Elective Colorectal Resection for Cancer. Ann Surg 2007, 245(6):867-72.

[28] Muller S, Zalunardo MP,Hubner M et al: A fast-track program reduces complications and length of hospital stay after open colonic surgery. Gastroenterology 2009;136: 842-7

[29] Serclova Z, Dytrych P, Marvan J et al: Fast-track in open intestinal surgery: prospective randomized study (Clinical Trials Gov Identifier no. NCT00123456). Clin Nutr 2009; 28(6): 618-24.
[30] Wind J, Hofland J, Preckel B et al: Perioperative strategy in colonic surgery: LAparoscopi and/or FAst track multimodal management versus standard care (LAFA trial). BMC Surgery 2006; 6(16): 1-8.
[31] Varadhan KK, Neal KR, Fearon KC et al: The enhanced recovery after surgery (ERAS) pathway for patients undergoing major elective open colorectal surgery: A meta-analysis of randomizes controlled trials. Clin Nutr 2010; 29: 434-40.
[32] Gustafsson UO, Hausel J, Thorell A et al: Adherence to the Enhanced Recovery After Surgery Protocol and Outcomes After Colorectal Cancer Surgery. Arch Surg 2011; Vol 146 (5): 571-7.
[33] Varadhan KK, Neal KR, Dejong CHC et al: Author's reply to letter from Dr. Gatt and colleagues. Clin Nutr 2010; Vol 29 (5): 691-2
[34] Spanjersberg WR, Reurings J, Keus F et al: Fast track surgery versus conventional recovery strategies for colorectal surgery. Cochrane Database Syst Rev 2011, CD007635.
[35] Eskicioglu C, Forbes SS, Aarts MA et al: Enhanced recovery after surgery (ERAS) programs for patients having colorectal surgery: a meta-analysis of randomized trials. J Gastrointest Surg 2009; Dec:13(12): 2321-9.
[36] Adamina M, Kehlet H, Tomlinson GA et al: Enhanced recovery pathways optimize health outcomes and resource utilization: a meta-analysis of randomized controlled trials in colorectal surgery. Surgery 2011; Jun; 149(6):830-40.
[37] Sutton AJ & Abrams KR: Bayesian methods in meta-analysis and evidence synthesis. Med Res 2001; Vol 10(4): 277-303.
[38] Ljungqvist O, Nygren J, Thorell A et al: Preoperative nutrition – elective surgery in the fed or the overnight fasted state. Clin Nutr 2001; 20 (Supplement 1): 167-71.
[39] Thorell A, Nygren J & Ljungqvist O: Insulin resistance: a marker of surgical stress. Curr Opin Clin Nutr Metab Care. 1999 Jan; 2(1):69-78.
[40] Nygren J, Soop M, Thorell A et al: Preoperative oral carbohydrate administration reduces postoperative insulin resistance. Clin Nutr 1998; 17:65-71.
[41] Langelotz C, Spies C, Müller JM et al: "Fast-track"-Rehabilitation in Surgery, a Multimodal Concept. Acta chir belg 2005; 105:555-9.
[42] Pasero C & Belden J: Evidence-Based Perianesthesia Care: Accelerated Postoperative Recovery Programs. J Perianaesth Nurs 2006;21(3):168-76.
[43] Lassen K, Soop M, Nygren J et al: Consensus Review of Optimal Perioerative Care in Colorectal Suregery. Arch Surg 2009;144(10): 961-9.
[44] Wilmore DW & Kehlet H: Management of patients in fast track surgery. Clin Rev 2001; Feb (322): 473-6.
[45] Archer SB, Burnett RJ, Flesch LV et al: Implementation of a clinical pathway decreases length of stay and hospital charges for patients undergoing total colectomy and ileal pouch/ anal anastomosis. Am J Surg. 2005 Mar;189(3):268-72
[46] Mohn AC, Bernardshaw SV, Ristesund SM et al: Enhanced recovery after colorectal surgery. Results from a prospective observational two-centre study. Scand J Surg 2009;98: 155-9.

[47] Wind J, Polle SW, Fung Kon JinPHP et al: Systematic review of enhanced recovery programmes in colonic surgery. Br J Surg 2006; 93: 800–809
[48] Pritts TA, Nussbaum MS, Flesh LV et al: Implementation of a Clinical Pathway Decreases Length of Stay and Cost for Bowel Resection. Ann Surg 1999; 230(5): 728-33.
[49] Kehlet H & Holte K: Effect of postoperative analgesia on surgical outcome Br. J. Anaesth., July 1, 2001; 87(1): 62 - 72.
[50] MacKay G, Fearon K, McConnachie A et al: Randomized clinical trial of the effect of postoperative intravenous fluid restriction on recovery after elective colorectal surgery. Br J Surg 2006; 93: 1469–74.
[51] Ramirex JM, Blasco JA, Roig JV et al: Enhanced recovery in colorectal surgery: a multicentre study. BMC Surgery 2011;11:1-8.
[52] Halsted WS. Circular suture of the intestine: an experimental study. Am J Med Sci 1887; 94: 436-61.
[53] Hughes ESR: Asepsis in large-bowel surgery. Ann Roy Coll Surg Engl 1972; Vol 51: 347-56.
[54] Irving AD & Scrimgeour D: Mechanical bowel preparation for colonic resection and anastomosis. Br J Surg 1987; Jul 74(7): 580-1.
[55] Burke P, Mealy K, Gillen P et al: Requirement for bowel preparation in colorectal surgery. Br J Surg 1994; Jun 81(6): 907-10.
[56] Platell C & Hall J: What is the role of bowel preparation in patients undergoing colorectal surgery? Dis Colon Rectum 1998; Vol42: 875-82.
[57] Contant CME, Hop WCJ, Van´t Sant HP et al: Mechanical bowel preparation for elective colorectal surgery: a multicenter randomised trial. Lancet 2007; 370: 2112-7.
[58] Jung B, Pahlman L, Nystrom PO et al for the Mechanical Bowel Preparation Study Group. Multicentre randomized clinical trial of mechanical bowel preparation in elective colonic surgery. Br J Surg 2007; 94: 689-95.
[59] Slim K, Vicaut E, Panis Y et al: Meta-analysis of randomised clinical trials of colorectal surgery with or without mechanical bowel preparation. Br J Surg 204; 91: 1125-30.
[60] Guenaga KF, Matos D, Castro AA et al: Mechanical bowel preparation for elective colorectal surgery. Cochrane database Syst rev 2005; 1: CD001544.
[61] Guenaga KK, Matos D, & Wille-Jorgensen P: Mechanical bowel preperation for elective colorectal surgery. Cochrane Database Syst Rev 2011; (1):CD001544.
[62] Lichtenstein G: Bowel preparations for colonoscopy: a review. Am J Health Syst Pharm. 2009 Jan 1; 66(1):27-37.
[63] Hoy SM, Scott LJ & Wagstaff AJ: Sodium picosulfate/magnesium citrate: a review of its use as a colorectal cleanser. Drugs. 2009; 69(1):123-36.
[64] Belsey J, Epstein O & Heresbach D: Systematic review: adverse event reports for oral sodium phosphate and polyethylene glycol. Aliment Pharmacol Ther. 2009 Jan;29(1):15-28.
[65] Dykes C & Cash BD: Key safety issues of bowel preparations for colonoscopy and importance of adequate hydration. Gastroenterol Nurs. 2008 Jan-Feb; 31(1):30-5; quiz 36-7.
[66] Wexner SD, Beck DE, Baron TH et al: A consensus document on bowel preparation before colonoscopy: prepared by a Task Force from the American Socisty of Colon and Rectal Surgeons (ASCRS), the American Societu for Gastrointestinal

Endoscopy (ASGE), and the Society of American Gastrointestinal and Endoscopic Surgeons (SAGES). Surh Endosc 2006; Vol 20(7): 1161.
[67] Lewis SJ, Egger M, Sylvester PA et al: Early enteral feeding versus "nil by mouth" after gastrointestinal surgery: systematic review and meta-analysis of controlled trials. BMJ 2001;323:773-6
[68] Smedley F, Bowling T, James M et al: Randomized clinical trial of the effects of preoperative and postoperative oral nutritional supplements on clinical course and cost of care. Br J Surg. 2004 Aug; 91(8):983-90.
[69] Snow J: Fatal Application of Chloroform. Lancet 1848; (1): 161-2
[70] Snow J: On Chloroform and other Anaesthetics, ed. Richardson BW. London: Churchill, 1858.
[71] Hall CC: Aspiration pneumonitis An obstetric hazard. JAMA 1940; 114: 928-33.
[72] Fasting S, Soreide E & Raeder: Changing preoperative fasting policies. Acta Anaesthesiol Scand 1998; 42: 1188-91.
[73] Kaska M, Grosmanová T, Havel E et al: The impact and safety of preoperative oral or intravenous carbohydrate administration versus fasting in colorectal surgery--a randomized controlled trial. Wien Klin Wochenschr. 2010 Jan;122 (1-2):23-30.
[74] Ljungqvist O, Nygren J, Hausel J et al: Preoperative nutrition therapy - novel developments. Scand J Nutr 2000; Vol 44: 3-7.
[75] Brady MC, Kinn S, Stuart P et al: Preoperative fasting for adults to prevent perioperative complications. Cochrane Database Syst Rev 2003; Issue 4: CD004423.
[76] Nygren J, Thorell A, Jacobsson H et al: Preoperative gastric emptying: Effect of anxiety and oral carbohydrate administration. Ann Surg 1995; 222:728-34.
[77] Ljungqvist O, Thorell A, Gutniak M et al: Glucose infusion instead of preoperative fasting reduces postoperative insulin resistance. J Am Coll Surg 1994; 178: 329-36.
[78] Andersen HK, Lewis SJ & Thomas S: Early enteral nutrition within 24h of colorectal surgery versus later commencement of feeding for postoperative complications. Cochrane Database Syst Rev 2006; Issue 4: CD004080.
[79] Hausel J, Nygren J, Lagerkranser M et al: A Carbohydrate-Rich Drink Reduces Preoperative Discomfort in Elective Surgery Patients. Anesth Analg. 2001 Nov;93(5):1344-50.
[80] Noblett SE, Watson DS, Houng H et al: Pre-operative oral carbohydrate loading in colorectal surgery: a randomized controlled trial. Colorectal Dis 2006; 8: 563-9.
[81] Rosenberg J & Harvald T: Severe Complications with Diclofenak After Colonic Resection. Dis Colon Rectum 2007; 50 (5): 685. (Letter)
[82] Wolff BG, Michelassi F, Gerkin TM et al: Alvimopan, a Novel, Peripherally Acting μ Opioid Antagonist. Ann Surg 2004; Vol 240(4): 728-35.
[83] Delaney CP, Wolff BG, Viscusi ER et al: Alvimopan, for PostoperativeIleus Following Bowel Resection. Ann Surg 2007; Vol 245(3): 355-63.
[84] Bisgaard T, Klarskov B, Kehlet H et al: Preoperative Dexamethasone Improves Surgical Outcome After Laparoscopic Cholecystectomy. Ann Surg 2003; Vol 238(5): 651-60.
[85] Srinivasa S, Kahokehr AA, Yu TC et al: Preoperative Glucocorticoid Use in Major Abdominal Surgery: Systematic Review and Meta-Analysis of Randomized Trials. Ann Surg 2011; Aug; 254(2): 183-91.

[86] Fukami Y, Terasaki M, Okamoto Y et al: Efficacy of preoperative dexamethasone in patients with laparoscopic cholecystectomy: a prospective randomized double-blind study. J Hepatobiliary Pancreat Surg. 2009;16(3):367-71. Epub 2009 Mar 31.
[87] Kirdak T, Yilmazlar A, Cavun S et al: Does single, low-dose preoperative dexamethasone improve outcomes after colorectal surgery based on an enhanced recovery protocol? Double-blind, randomized clinical trial. Am Surg. 2008 Feb;74(2):160-7.
[88] Zargar-Shostari K, Sammour T, Kahokehr A et al: Randomised clinical trial of the effect of glucocorticoids on peripheral inflammation and postoperative recovery after colectomy. Br J Surg 2009; 96: 1253-61.
[89] O'Donnell M & Weitz JI: Thromboprophylaxis in surgical patients. Can J Surg 2003; Vol 46(2): 129-35.
[90] Bergqvist D: Low molecular weight heparin for the prevention of venous thromboembolism after abdominal surgery. Br J Surg 2004; 91: 965-74.
[91] Leonardi MJ, McGory ML & Ko CY: A Systematic Review of Deep Venous Thrombosis Prophylaxis in Cancer Patients: Implications for Improving Quality. Ann Surg Onc 2007; Vol 14(2): 929-936.
[92] Geerts WH, Bergqvist D, Pineo GF et al: : Prevention of Venous Thromboembolism: American College of Chest Physicians Evidence-Based Clinical Practice Guidelines (8th edition). Chest 2008; 133; 381-453.
[93] Mohn AC, Egge J, Røkke O: Low Risk of Thromboembolic Complications after Fast-Track Abdominal Surgery With Thrombosis-Prophylaxis Only During Hospital Stay. Gastroenterology Research Vol. 4, No. 3, Jun 2011.
[94] Rasmussen MS, Jorgensen LN, Wille-Jorgensen P et al: Prolonged prophylaxis with dalteparin to prevent late thromboembolic complications in patients undergoing major abdominal surgery: a multicenter randomized open-label study. Thromb Haemost 2006; 4: 2384–2390.
[95] Kakkar VV, Cohen AT, Edmonson RA: Low molecular weight versus standard heparin for prevention of venous thromboembolism after major abdominal surgery. The Thromboprophylaxis Collaborative Group. Lancet. 1993 Jan 30;341(8840):259-65.
[96] Vaitkus PT, Leizorovicz A, Cohen AT: Mortality rates and risk factors for asymptomatic deep vein thrombosis in medical patients. Thromb Haemost. 2005 Jan;93(1):76-9.
[97] Wille-Jørgensen P, Jorgensen LN, Crawford M: Asymptomatic postoperative deep vein thrombosis and the development of postthrombotic syndrome. A systematic review and meta-analysis. Thromb Haemost. 2005 Feb; 93(2):236-41.
[98] ENOXACAN Study Group: Efficacy and safety of enoxaparin versus unfractionated heparin for prevention of deep vein thrombosis in elective cancer surgery: a double-blind randomized multicentre trial with venographic assessment. Br J Surg 1997; 84(8):1099-1103.
[99] Rasmussen MS, Jørgensen LN, Wille-Jørgensen P: Prolonged thromboprophylaxis with Low Molecular Weight heparin for abdominal or pelvic surgery. Cochrane Database Syst Rev 2009; Issue 1: CD004318.
[100] Bergqvist D, Agnelli G, Cohen AT et al: The ENOXACAN II investigators: Duration of prophylaxis against venous thromboembolism with enoxaparin after surgery for cancer. NEJM 2002; 346: 975-80.

[101] Wille-Jørgensen P, Rasmussen MS, Andersen BR et al: Heparins and mechanical methods for thromboprophylaxis in colorectal surgery. Cochrane Database Syst Rev 2009, Issue 1: CD004318.
[102] Raahave D, Hansen OH, Carstensen HE et al: Septic wound complications after whole bowel irrigation before colorectal operations. Acta Chir Scand. 1981; 147(3):215-8.
[103] Baum ML, Anish DS, Chalmers TC et al: A Survey of Clinical Trials of Antibiotic Prophylaxis in Colon Surgery: Evidence against Further Use of No-Treatment Controls. NEJM 1981; 305: 795-9.
[104] Nelson RL, Glenny AM & Song F: Antimicrobial prophylaxis for colorectal surgery. Cochrane Database Syst Rev 2009; CD001181.
[105] Should antimicrobial prophylaxis in colorectal surgery include agents effective against both anaerobic and aerobic microorganisms? A double-blind, multicenter study. The Norwegian Study Group for Colorectal Surgery. Surgery. 1985 Apr; 97(4):402-8.
[106] Giercksky K-E, Danielsen S, Garberg O et al: A Single Dose Tinidazole and Doxycycline Prophylaxis in Elective Surgery of Colon and Rectum. A Prospective Controlled Clinical Multicenter Study. Ann Surg 1982; Feb: 227-31.
[107] Bradshaw BG, Liu SS, Thirlby RC: Standardized Perioperative Care Protocols and Reduced Length of Stay After Colon Surgery. J Am Coll Surg 1998
[108] Carli F, Trudel JL, Belliveau P. The effect of intraoperative thoracic epidural anesthesia and postoperative analgesia on bowel function after colorectal surgery: a prospective, randomized trial. Dis Colon Rectum 2001;44: 1083-1089.
[109] Moraca RJ, Sheldon DG & Thirlby RC: The Role of Epidural Anesthesia and Analgesia in Surgical Practice. Ann Surg 2003; Vol 238(5): 663-73.
[110] Jorgensen H, Wetterslev J and Moiniche S et al., Epidural local anaesthetics versus opioid-based analgesic regimens on postoperative gastrointestinal paralysis, PONV and pain after abdominal surgery, Cochrane Database Syst Rev 2001: Issue 4: CD001893.
[111] Zutshi M, Delaney CP, Senagore AJ et al: Randomized controlled trial comparing the controlled rehabilitation with early ambulation and diet pathway versus the controlled rehabilitation with early ambulation and diet with preemptive epidural anesthesia/analgesia after laparotomy and intestinal resection. Am J Surg 2005, Mar189(3):268-72.
[112] Rigg JR, Jamrozik K, Myles PS et al: Epidural anaesthesia and analgesia and outcome of major surgery: a randomised trial. Lancet. 2002; Vol 359(9314):1276-82.
[113] Ahmed J, Lim M, Khan S et al: Predictors of length of stay in patients having elective colorectal surgery within an enhanced recovery protocol. Int J Surg 2010; 8(8): 628-32.
[114] Kariv Y, Delaney CP, Senagore AJ et al: Clinical outcomes and cost analysis of a "fast-track" postoperative care pathway for ileal pouch-anal anastomosis. A case control study. Dis Colon Rectum 2007; 50(2):137-46.
[115] Apfel CC, Korttila K, Abdalla M et al: A Factorial Trial of Six Interventions for the Prevention of Postopertive Nausea and Vomiting. NEJM 2004; 350(24): 2441-51.
[116] Apfel CC & Roewer N: Postoerpative nausea and vomiting. Anaesthesist 2004; 53(4): 377-89.

[117] Lindgren PG, Nordgren SR, Oresland T et al: Midline or transverse abdominal incision for right-sided colon cancer: a randimized trial. Colorectal Dis 2001; 3:46-50.

[118] Reza MM, Blasco JA, Andradas E et al: Systematic review of laparoscopic versus open surgery for colorectal cancer. Br J Surg 2006; 93: 921–928

[119] Delaney CP, Marcello PW, Sonoda T et al: Gastrointestinal recovery after laparoscopic colectomy: results of a prospective, observational, multicenter study. Surg Endosc 2010; 24: 653-61.

[120] Senagore AJ, Duepree HJ, Delaney CP et al: Results of a standardized technique and postoperative care plan for laparoscopic sigmoid colectomy: a 30-month experience. Dis Colon Rectum. 2003 Apr;46(4):503-9.

[121] Raue W, Haase O, Junghans Tet al: "Fast-track" multimodal rehabilitation program improves outcome after laparoscopic sigmoidectomy A controlled prospective evaluation Surg Endosc (2004) 18: 1463–1468

[122] Schwenk W, Haase O Neudecker JJ et al: Short term benefits for laparoscopic colorectal resection. Cochrane Database Syst Rev 2005; Issue 3: CD003145.

[123] King PM, Blazeby JM, Ewings P et al: Randomized clinical trial comparing laparoscopic and open surgery for colorectal cancer within an enhanced recovery programme. Br J Surg 2006; 93: 300–308.

[124] Callery MP: Preoperative Steroids for Laparoscpic Surgery. Ann Surg 2003; Vol 238(5): 661-2.

[125] Wangensteen OH & Paine JR: Treatment of acute intestinal obstruction by suction with the duodenal tube. JAMA 1933; 101(20):1532-1539.

[126] Cheatham ML, Chapman WC, Key SP et al: A Meta-Analysis of Selective Versus Routine Nasogastric Decompression After Elective Laparotomy. Ann Surg 1995; Vol 221(5): 469-78.

[127] Verma R & Nelson RL: Prophylactic nasogastric decompression after abdominal surgery. Cochrane Database Syst Rev 2007; Issue 3: CD004929.

[128] Olesen KL, Birch M, Bardram L et al: Value of nasogastric tube after colorectal surgery. Acta Chir Scand. 1984;150(3):251-3.

[129] Nelson R, Edwards S & Tse B: Prophylactic nasogastric decompression after abdominal surgery. Cochrane Database Syst Rev 2007; Issue 3: CD004929.

[130] Shires T, Williams J & Brown F: Acute Change in Extracellular Fluids Associatied with Major Surgical Procedures. Ann Surg 1961; Nov: 803-10.

[131] Nielsen OM & Engell HC. Changes in extracellular sodium content after elective abdominal vascular surgery. Acta Chir Scand 1986; 152:587-91.

[132] Mecrey PM, Barden RP & Ravdis IS: Nutritial edema: its effect on the gastric emptying time before and after gastric operations. Surgery 1937; 1: 53-64.

[133] Lobo DN, Bostock KA, Neal KR et al: Effect of salt and water balance on recovery of gastrointestinal function after elective colonic resection: a randomised controlled trial. Lancet 2002; 359(May):1812-18.

[134] More FD: Metabolic Care of the Surgical Patient. Philadelphia: WB Saubders Co 1959.

[135] Holte K, Sharrock NE & Kehlet H: Pathophysiology and clinical implications of perioperative fluid excess. Br J Ane 2002; 89(4):622-32.

[136] Tambyraja AL, Sengupta F, MacGregor AB et al: Patterns and clinical outcomes associated with routine intravenous sodium and fluid administration after colorectal resection. World J Surg 2004;28: 1046-51.

[137] Brandstrup B,Tønnesen H, Beier-Holgersen R et al: Effects of Intravenous Fluid Restriction on Postoperative Complications: Comparison of Two Perioperative Fluid Regimens. Ann Surg 2003;238: 641–648)
[138] Varadhan KK & Lobo DN: A meta-analysis of randomised controlled trials of intravenous fluid therapy in major alective open abdominal surgery: getting the balance right. Proc Nutr Soc 2010; 69(4): 48-98.
[139] Vermeulen H, Hofland J, Lagamate DA et al: Intravenous fluid restriction after major abdominal surgery: a randomized blinded clinical trial. Trials 2009; 10(50): 1-11.
[140] Srinivasa S, Taylor MH, Sammour T et al: Oesophageal Doppler-guided fluid administration in colorectal surgery: critical appraisal of published clinical trials. Acta Anaesthesiol Scand 2011; Jan; 55(1): 4-13.
[141] Rahbari NN, Zimmermann JB, Schmidt T et al: Meta-analysis of standard, restrictive and supplemental fluid administration in colorectal surgery. Br J Surg 2009;96(4):331-41.
[142] Karliczek A, Jesus EC, Matos D et al: Drainage or nondrainage in elective colorectal anastomosis: a systematic review and meta-analysis. Colorectal Dis 2006; 8: 259-65.
[143] Petrowsky H, Demartines N, Rousson V et al: Evidence-based Value of Prophylactic Drainage in Gastrointestinal Surgery. Ann Surg 2004; Vol 240(6): 1074-85.
[144] Sims FM: Case of Ovariotomy Successfully Performed during Suppurative Peritonitis and Pyæmic Fever: with Remarks. BMJ 1879 May 24; 1(960): 771–772.
[145] Sagar PM, Couse N, Kerin M et al: Randomized trial of drainage of colorectal anastomosis. Br J Surg. 1993 Jun; 80(6):769-71.
[146] Sagar PM, Hartley MN, MacFie J et al: Randomized trial of pelvic drainage after rectal resection. Dis Colon Rectum. 1995 Mar; 38(3):254-8.
[147] Urbach DR, Kennedy ED & Cohen MM: Colon and Rectal Anastomosis Do Not Require Routine Drainage. Ann Surg 1999; Vol 229(2): 174-80.
[148] Jesus EC, Karliczek A, Matos D et al: Prophylactic anastomotic drainage for colorectal surgery. Cochrane Database Syst Rev 2004; Issue 4: CD002100.
[149] Harms B & Heise CP: Pharmacologic Management of Postoperative Ileus. The Next Chapter I GI Surgery. Ann Surg 2007; Vol 245(3): 364-5 (ed.)
[150] Reissman P, Teoh TA, Cohen SM et al: Is Early Oral Feeding Safe After Elective Colorectal Surgery?A Prospective Randomized Trial. AnnSurg 1995,222(1): 73-77
[151] Binderow SR, Cohen SM, Wexner SD et al: Must early postoperative oral intake be limited to laparoscopy? Dis Colon Rectum 1994; 37(6): 584-9.
[152] Carr CS, Ling KDE, Boulos P et al: Randomised trial of safety and afficacy of immediate postoperative enteral feeding in patients undergoing gastrointestinal resection. BMJ 1996; Vol 312: 869-71.
[153] Schoetz DJ Jr, Bockler M, Rosenblatt MS et al: "Ideal" length of stay after colectomy: whose ideal? Dis Colon Rectum 1997; 40: 806-810.
[154] Di Fronzo LA, Cymerman J & O¨Connell TX: Factors affecting early postoperative feeding following elective open colon resection. Arch Surg 1999; 134(9): 941-6.
[155] Lewis SJ, Andersen HK & Thomas S: Early enteral nutrition within 24h of intestinal surgery versus later commencement of feeding: a systematic review and meta-analysis. J Gastroint Surg 2009; Mar: 13(3): 569-75.

[156] Sammour T, Zargar-Shoshtari K, Bhat A et al: A programme of Enhanced Recovery After Surgery (ERAS) is a cost-effective intervention in elective colonic surgery. NZMJ 2010; 123(1319): 61-70.
[157] King PM, Blazeby JM, Ewings P et al: The influence of an Enhanced Recovery Programme on clinical outcomes, costs and quality of life after surgery for colorectal cancer. Colorectal Dis 2006; Vol 8(6): 506-13.
[158] Kehlet H: Fast-track colorectal surgery. Lancet 2008: Vol 371: 791-3.
[159] Stephen AE & Berger DL: Shortened length of stay and hospital cost reduction with implementation of an accelerated clinical care pathway after elective colon resection. Surgery 2003; Mar; 133(3): 277-82.
[160] Lassen K, Hannemann P, Ljungqvist O et al: Patterns in current perioperative practice: survey of colorectal surgeons in five northern European countries. BMJ 2005;330:1420–1
[161] Grol R & Grimshaw J; From best evidence to best practice: effective implementation of change in patient's care. Lancet. 2003 Oct 11; 362(9391):1225-30.

2

Postoperative Ileus in Elective Colorectal Surgery: Management Strategies

J. Ahmed, S. Mehmood and J. MacFie
Scarborough General Hospital, Scarborough
United Kingdom

1. Introduction

Postoperative ileus (POI) is a condition characterised by transient interruption of gut function following surgical intervention. Ileus develops due to impaired motility of the gastrointestinal tract in the absence of any mechanical bowel obstruction (Holte and Kehlet 2000). This results in disturbance of coordinated propulsive action leading to accumulation of luminal gas and fluid mainly within small bowel. Clinically it is manifested by abdominal distension, nausea, vomiting and diet intolerance (Lubawski and Saclarides 2008; Parvizi, et al. 2008).

Despite a number of advances in perioperative care and surgical techniques, POI remains one of the commonest challenges in surgery. Although most commonly seen following abdominal surgery, it is also associated with extra-abdominal operations such as cardiothoracic and orthopaedic procedures (Parvizi, et al. 2008; Stewart and Waxman 2010). Historically, POI has been regarded as an inevitable event after major abdominal surgery and it is considered the single largest factor prolonging the length of hospital stay (LOS) following gastrointestinal surgery (Lubawski and Saclarides 2008). It impacts greatly on patient's recovery even after uncomplicated abdominal surgery. Similarly, postoperative ileus is one of the commonest factors affecting healthcare costs in surgical patients. Furthermore, POI causes significant frustration amongst the patients and the surgeons alike (Asgeirsson, et al. 2010).

In recent years, some progress has been made in understanding of underlying causative mechanisms of POI. The multifaceted pathophysiology of POI includes neurogenic, hormonal, inflammatory and pharmacological factors which have been targeted to reduce the incidence and duration of POI. However, there is no definitive treatment to prevent this condition. Key principles in the prevention and management of POI pertain to minimising surgical trauma and preserving normal physiological functions, including gut function. Evidence suggests that this is best achieved by a multimodal approach involving a host of interventions in the perioperative period. Perhaps the most significant development in recent times is the formulation of enhanced recovery after surgery (ERAS) protocols. ERAS protocols provide a multimodal approach to optimising perioperative care and enhancing postoperative recovery. Likewise, minimally invasive surgery i.e. laparoscopic approach has been shown to provide benefits like reduction in length of stay in hospital. Similarly, newer pharmacological therapies (e.g. Mu-opioid receptor antagonist) have shown promising results, however, more scientific evidence is awaited in this area.

In this chapter, we give an account of pathophysiology, natural history, and classification of ileus. Different strategies to prevent and manage POI such as ERAS protocols, minimally invasive surgery and pharmacological approaches are discussed.

2. History and definitions of POI

Ileus is a Greek word which literally means "obstructed" however it is referred to as a functional impediment without mechanical obstruction. POI has been a recognised condition for more than two centuries. The exact definition of POI has been a topic for debate for over a century. It was suggested by Finney in 1906 to divide the phenomnon of ileus into pathophysiological, mechanical, septic or adynamic ileus (Finney 1906). One hundred years later in 2006, the '*Postoperative Ileus Management Council' (PIMC)* was formed by experts in the field of surgery and anaesthesia. The PIMC collected all scientific evidence and developed a consensus on the definition of POI. According to this panel POI is a:

"transient cessation of coordinated bowel motility after surgical intervention, which prevents effective transit of intestinal contents or tolerance of oral intake".

The PIMC categorised POI into primary and secondary ileus. Primary POI develops in the absence of any precipitating factors (i.e. absence of any complications), while secondary POI develops in the presence of a complication such as wound infection, intra-abdominal collection, anastomotic leak, and sepsis etc. In addition, a further three types of POI were described based on the part of gastrointestinal tract (GIT) involved. Type–I POI involves all part of the GIT and thus called pan-intestinal ileus. Clinically it is manifested as nausea and vomiting along with absence of bowel movement or passage of flatus. Type–II POI affects only the upper GIT and manifests as nausea and vomiting. These patients are able to tolerate food but are unable to pass flatus. Type–III POI comprises of ileus of the lower GIT. The patients may be able to tolerate food but are unable to pass flatus or have a bowel motion (Delaney C 2006).

The duration of POI and the cardinal features of its resolution are important aspects which need careful consideration. The minimum time period following surgery before ileus develops is not well defined. Animal and human models have shown that return of gut function occurs first of all in small bowel (24 hours) followed by stomach (48 hours) and colon (48 to 72 hours) (Lubawski and Saclarides 2008). It has been suggested that the colon may take up to 120 hours to resume normal peristaltic activities postoperatively. (Miedema and Johnson 2003).

The return of gut function is historically assessed by either of the presence of bowel sounds, passage of flatus or stool, or tolerance to oral food. Passage of flatus or stool and/or presence of bowel sounds are considered as the benchmark criteria for the recovery of bowel function. However, concerns have been expressed about the validity and accuracy in recording these signs. For example, presence of bowel sounds does not necessarily indicate return of propulsive activities of the whole bowel as they may only represent small bowel activity without colonic peristalsis (Holte and Kehlet 2000). In addition, accuracy of recording these features is usually low. To record presence of bowel sounds requires frequent auscultation which is practically difficult. Similarly, passage of flatus is also not the ideal end point. Some patients are simply not comfortable to report it whereas others may not be able to recall passing flatus in the postoperative peroid. The passage of stool is also considered to have low specificity. A patient might report having a bowel movement which would be representing distal bowel evacuation as opposed to global gastrointestinal tract function. Hence determination of the end of postoperative ileus is another contentious issue.

The combination of all three signs (i.e. presence of bowel sounds, passage of stool or flatus along with tolerance of oral feed) provides higher accuracy in confirming resolution of POI. Thus, based on the available evidence and PIMC consensus report the resolution of POI can be defined:

"the duration of POI is the time from the surgery until passage of stool or flatus and until oral feed that is tolerated and maintained during 24 hours".

However, it is important to appreciate that uncertainties in criteria for the resolution of POI have impact on the conclusions of various studies published in the literature (Boeckxstaens and de Jonge 2009).

3. Pathophysiology of post-operative ileus

3.1 Normal physiology

The normal motility of gut is maintained by the complex interaction among the central nervous system, enteric nervous system, and hormonal and local factors directly acting on the intestinal smooth muscle (Livingston and Passaro 1990; Mattei and Rombeau 2006). The autonomic nerve system consists of parasympathetic, sympathetic and enteric nervous systems. It has a profound effect on gut motility, ion transportation and is involved in secretory and absorptive processes within GIT. The parasympathetic part of the nervous system is provided by vagus (proximal GIT) and pelvic parasympathetic (distal GIT) nerves. These nerve fibres have a stimulating effect on GIT. The sympathetic innervation is provided by the splanchnic nerve. These post-ganglionic fibres run along the arteries and synapse with the myenteric plexus on the gut wall. The sympathetic nerve fibres have an inhibitory effect on gut which includes inhibition of secretions and motility, and constriction of sphincters and blood vessels. The animal models have shown the sympathetic control is dominant over parasympathetic (Livingston and Passaro 1990).

The enteric nervous system, which is also known as the intrinsic nervous system, consists of myenteric and submucosal plexuses. It makes an important contribution in controlling GI motility and coordinating relaxation and contraction of smooth muscle. The myenteric plexus mainly controls motility of the digestive tract, whilst the submucosal plexus mainly regulates the gastrointestinal blood flow and epithelial function. The enteric nervous system consists of sensory, motor and interneurons. Acetylcholine is the major neurotransmitter which is produced by enteric neurons. Although, the enteric nervous system has the ability to function independently, for normal digestive process it links with the central (extrinsic) nervous system. Due to these cross connections gut provides sensory information to the central nervous system and therefore it may recieve efferent signals from it (Boeckxstaens and de Jonge 2009; Luckey, et al. 2003; Wood 2008). In addition, various hormones and enzymes play an important role in gut function and its motility. The gastrointestinal tract is the largest endocrine organ, called enteric endocrine system, with endocrine glands diffusely scattered throughout the GIT. The hormones secreted by these glands work by a negative feedback mechanism. The enteric endocrine system and nervous systems (enteric and autonomic nervous systems) work in a coordinated way to maintain the regular contractions of smooth muscle. It has two specific patterns: slow wave and spike potentials. The spike potentials are true action potentials which trigger the muscle contraction. The motility of stomach and small bowel varies according to fed and fasting states. Further, in fed state the number of contractions, their intensity and duration are based on the food ingested. During fasting state the migrating motor complex (MMC) dictates the pattern of bowel contraction (Luckey, et al. 2003). Due to MMC, the remnants of meal, bacterial and other debris are pushed into the large intestine. Hence they have housekeeping function and prevent bacterial overgrowth in the small intestine. Thus any imbalance in autonomic nerves system, enteric endocrine and the local environment may impair the normal gut motility and digestive process, and may lead to ileus.

3.2 Pathophysiology

Ileus is caused by temporary inhibition of extrinsic motility regulation and is more prominent in the colon, while paralytic ileus involves all or part of the GIT and is caused by the inhibition of local and intrinsic contractile systems along with extrinsic inhibition (Bauer and Boeckxstaens 2004). Hence each local factor, autonomic nervous system and hormonal effect has an independent role in the development of POI.

In the past, surgical stress was considered to cause POI by increasing serum catecholamine concentration which would inhibit the gut motility and augment sympathetic activity (Smith, et al. 1977). However, experiments on animal models have shown that although adrenalectomy reduces the level of catecholamine, it does not improve POI. In contrast, splanchnicectomy partially improves ileus (Dubois, et al. 1975). These findings support the hypothesis that the sympathetic nervous system is independent of adrenal activity in causing ileus (Livingston and Passaro 1990). Similarly, vasopressin inhibits intestinal motility (Mitchell and Collin 1985). It is released as a part of stress response following surgical trauma and after the use of opiates (Cochrane, et al. 1981); (Weiskopf, et al. 1987). The exact mechanism by which vasopressin mediates dysmotility is not clear. However, it is suggested that vasopressin is related to reduction in mesenteric blood flow which may subsequently cause impairment of gastrointestinal motility (Livingston and Passaro 1990).

Evidence suggests that three major mechanisms play important role in the development of POI, namely; neurogenic, inflammatory and pharmacological mechanisms. Either of these can cause ileus independently, as does their cumulative effect (Bauer and Boeckxstaens 2004).

3.2.1 Neurogenic mechanisms

In 1872, Golz suggested that intestinal contractility increases after division of the neural axis. This was one of the first observations suggesting the presence of inhibitory spinal reflexes (Bauer and Boeckxstaens 2004). Later evidence has shown that splanchnicectomy improves bowel contraction after laparotomy. It was further suggested that splanchnic afferents are largely involved during gastrointestinal surgery, rather than vagal afferents, leading to hypomotility after surgical intervention (Bauer and Boeckxstaens 2004).

Recent investigations found that different neural pathways are activated during abdominal surgery. Their pathways depend upon the part of GIT involved and the intensity of nociceptive stimulus. For instance, skin incision and laparotomy activate an adrenergic inhibitory pathway, which is a low threshold spinal reflex and reduces gut motility (Boeckxstaens, et al. 1999). Strong stimuli, such as manipulation of the intestine, may activate an additional high-threshold supraspinal pathway (Barquist, et al. 1996). The corticotrophin-releasing factor (CRF) also plays a central role in this pathway. CRF antagonist has been shown to prevent gastric ileus (Bonaz and Tache 1997). Along with these there are non-adrenergic, vagally mediated, inhibitory pathways triggered by intense stimulation of splanchnic afferent fibres (Boeckxstaens, et al. 1999). Animal models have shown that nitric oxide (NO) is a most potent neurotransmitter in non-adrenergic pathways (Boeckxstaens, et al. 1999; De Winter, et al. 1997). Similarly, vasoactive intestinal peptide (VIP) acts as an inhibitory neurotransmitter during surgical stress (Boeckxstaens, et al. 2000; De Winter, et al. 1998).

Other studies have shown that μ-opioid receptor agonists (e.g morphine) prolong the duration of POI and k-opioid receptor agonists, such as fedotosine, resolve ileus through a peripheral action on non-vagal sensory afferent (Gue, et al. 1989). It is suggested that activation of k-opioid receptors on splanchnic afferent reduces POI by decreasing visceral nociception and inhibitory reflexes. The neural mechanism is primarily activated during the first few hours after surgery and cannot account of POI that lasts for days (Holte and Kehlet 2000; Reissman, et al. 1996).

3.2.2 Inflammatory mechanisms

The inflammatory response develops mainly at a local level and is associated directly with the development of POI (Bauer and Boeckxstaens 2004). For this local inflammatory response, muscularis externa provides a unique immunological compartment containing a rich network of macrophages (Faussone-Pellegrini, et al. 1990; Mikkelsen 1995). These macrophages secrete a number of inflammatory mediators such as cytokines, nitric oxide (NO), prostaglandins, and defensins (Cicalese, et al. 1996; Kagan, et al. 1994). Surgical manipulation of bowel activates the macrophages in muscularis externa stimulating release of above inflammaotory mediators (Kalff 1999; Schwarz, et al. 2001).

Intestinal manipulation also provokes the release of tumour necrosis factor-α (TNF-α), monocyte chemotactic protein-1, interleukin-1b and interleukin-6. These pro-inflammatory cytokines up-regulate adhesion molecules, such as intercellular adhesion molecule-1 (ICAM-1). This molecular response expands to cellular level and recruits more leucocytes (monocytes and neutropils) into the muscularis externa that further release NO, cytokines, reactive oxygen intermediates and proteases (Kalff, et al. 1999). The role of NO and prostaglandins in the development of POI has been shown in pharmacological and genetic studies ((Kalff 1999; Schwarz, et al. 2001). There is strong association between neural and inflammatory mechanisms as discussed below.

3.2.2.1 Inflammatory-neuronal interaction

It is well established that intestinal manipulation mediates local inflammation which causes inhibition of smooth muscle function. The manipulation of the small bowel not only causes ileus in the small bowel, it is also linked with delayed gastric emptying (de Jonge, et al. 2003). This raises the question as to whether there is any other mechanism which affects motility distant from the site of inflammation or manipulation? Bauer and Boeckxstaens (2004), suggested that:

"One possible mechanism could be an interaction between the inflammatory milieu of the postoperative muscularis and primary afferent neuronal activity, triggering the neural inhibitory pathways".

Animal models show that the delay in gastric emptying is induced by intestinal manipulation which occurs through an inhibitory adrenergic pathway. Up-regulation of cyclooxygenase-2 (COX-2) releases prostaglandins that participate in local inflammation and the development of POI (Schwarz, et al. 2001). A number of experimental studies have suggested that prostaglandins act as neuromodulators and their levels increase significantly following surgery. Animal models treated with selective COX-2 inhibitors show a reduction in incidence of ileus. Based on the findings of such studies Bauer and Boeckxstaens (2004) also concluded that:

"the intestinal inflammation in response to bowel manipulation results in primary afferent activation, initiating subsequent inhibitory motor reflexes to the gut, and leading to postoperative intestinal gut dysfunction, with prostaglandins playing a crucial role".

Furthermore, intestinal manipulation activates mast cells which play a vital role in the development of inflammation. During surgery even a gentle manipulation of intestine triggers the release of mast cell mediators. The activated mast cells release potent pro-inflammatory mediators such as TNF-α, protease and histamine which contribute to the inflammatory response. In addition, these mediators recruit more leucocytes and up-regulate adhesion molecules, all taking part in inflammatory process (Kubes and Kanwar 1994; Wershil, et al. 1996). The activated mast cells briefly increase intestinal permeability resulting in translocation of bacteria and consequently activation of resident macrophages in the muscularis externa. An inhibitory adrenergic neural pathway is also activated which impairs the neuromuscular function of the distant part of intestine, explaining the generalised features of ileus (Boeckxstaens and de Jonge 2009). Studies have demostrated that mast cell stabilizers improve gastric emptying and reduce inflammatory response (de Jonge, et al. 2003). Hence mast cells and resident macrophages are mainly responsible for activation of the innate immune system, leading to an inflammatory response after intestinal manipulation.

3.2.3 Pharmacological mechanisms

There are two types of opiates: endogenous and exogenous. Both play an important role in gastrointestinal dysmotility. Both are simliar and exert their actions through same opoid receptors (Prasad and Matthews 1999). Overall, opiates have an inhibitory effect which leads to impairment in gut motility, its secretions, and the transport of fluid and electrolytes across the gut wall. Understandibly, such actions lead to a delay in gastric emptying and inhibition of intestinal peristalsis and the development of POI (Kurz and Sessler 2003). This phenomenon has been proven in a number of studies on animal and human models which have shown that δ and μ opioid agonists diminish peristalsis (Bauer, et al. 1991; Bauer AJ 1991).

There are three different types of opoid receptors: δ (delta), μ (mu) and κ (kappa). Opiates have a receptor-specific effect on intestine and hence they mainly affect μ- receptors on GIT, while it has less effect on other organs receptors such as the brain or spinal cord. This is why morphine has more of a constipating effect than an analgesic effect. The requirement of morphine is four times more likely to increase to have an analgesic effect than constipating effect (4:1 ratio) (Holte and Kehlet 2000; Kalff, et al. 1998). Therefore, when opiates are used repeatedly, patients develop a tolerance to analgesic effect but not to the side effects on GIT (Holte and Kehlet 2000). A prospective study performed by Cali and colleagues did not show any significant correlation between the length of incision and the dose of morphine taken. However, it suggested that the dose of morphine is directly related to the return of gut function (Cali, et al. 2000). Similarly, opiates bind to leucocytes and affect the immune system which slows down gut motility. They also facilitate NO synthesis which plays a significant part in the pathogenesis of POI. Release of various hormones also plays a role in the pathogenesis of ileus. For example, corticotrophin-releasing factor stimulates inflammatory mediators in the bowel (Tache, et al. 1993).

In summary, there are multiple factors which contribute to the pathogenesis of POI and major mechanisms include neurogenic, inflammatory, pharmacological and hormonal responses (figure 1).

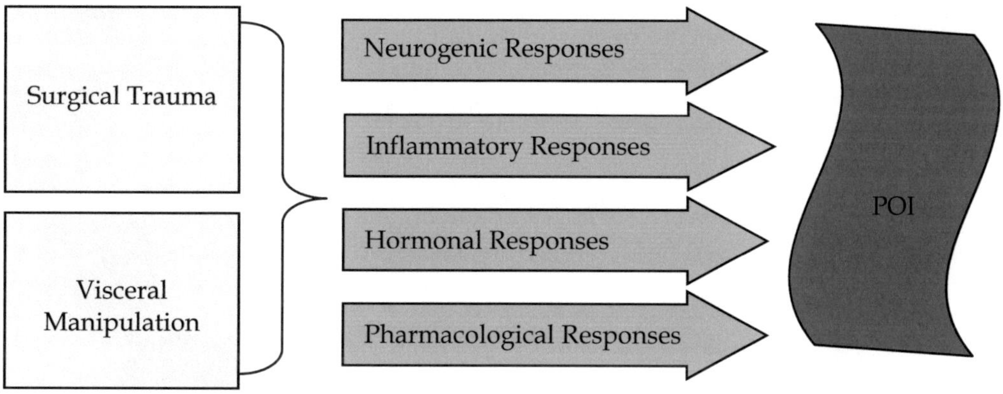

Fig. 1. Pathogenesis of post-operative ileus

4. Strategies to reduce POI

Over the past two decades, a number of strategies have been introduced to improve the quality of peroperative care. Most of those were primarily directed at reducing perioperative mortality, morbidity and LOS in hospital. All of those were aimed to prevent ileus by minimising the stress response and maintaining the normal body physiology during and after surgery. These include ERAS programmes, laparoscopic surgical approaches and the use of specific pharmaceutical agents. In this section, different strategies to prevent and manage POI are discussed.

4.1 Modalities to manage POI

4.1.1 Enhanced Recovery After Surgery (ERAS) protocols

ERAS protocols involve a series of measures taken pre-, per- and post-operatively which collectively ease the stress response to surgical trauma and enhance post-operative recovery. It has been shown that this 'multimodal rehabilitation' programme improves surgical outcome and patient satisfaction after elective surgery (Khoo, et al. 2007; Varadhan, et al. 2010; Wind, et al. 2006b). ERAS programme consists of a number of elements which are summarised in Figure- 2.

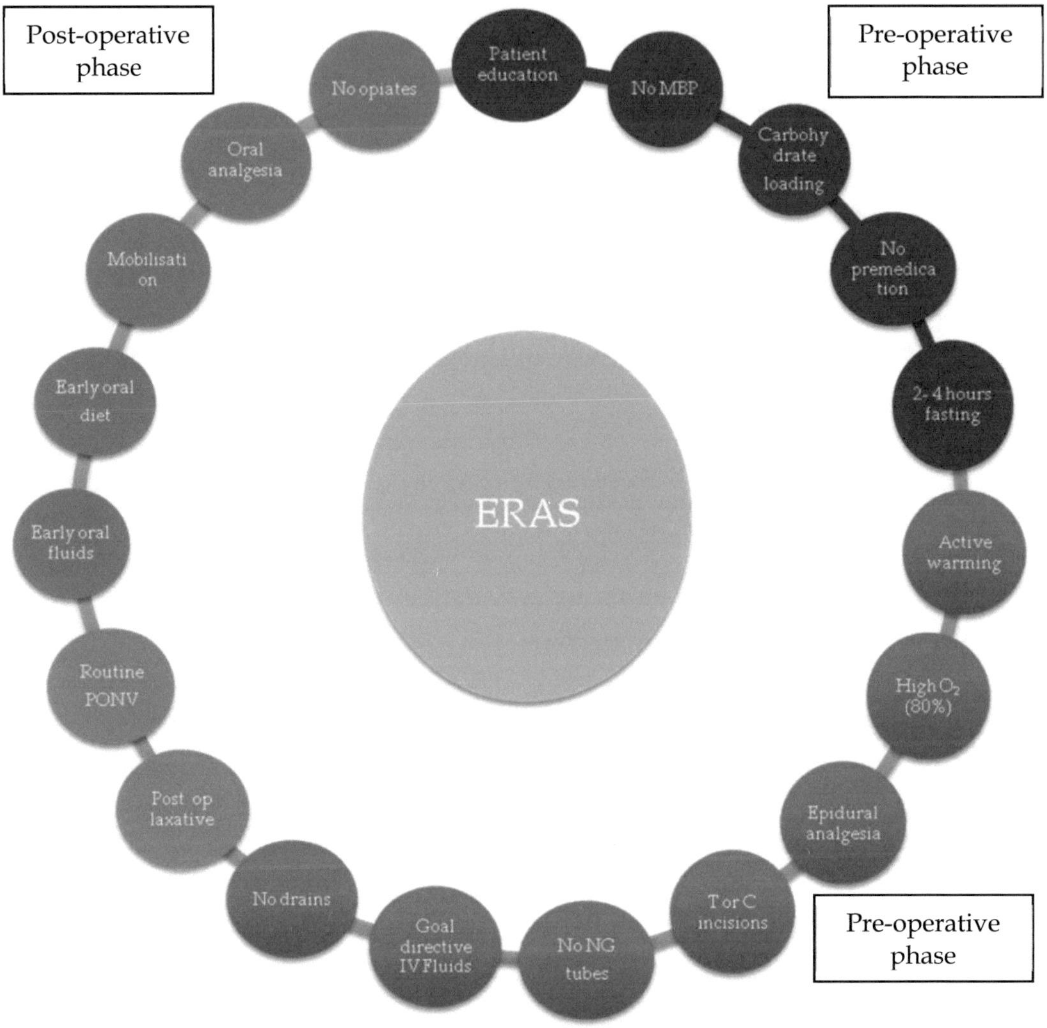

Fig. 2. MBP- Mechanical Bowel Preparation, T and C- Transverse and curve , NG- Nasogastric, PONV- prevention of nausea and vomiting. (Authors previously published this figure as Ahmed J et al, Colorectal Disease, 2011 Oct 11. doi: 10.1111/j.1463- 5 1318.2011.02856.x.)

4.1.2 Pre-operative components of ERAS protocols

Preoperative patient counselling and education prior to surgery is important aspect of ERAS protocols. Along with counselling, patients should also see other members of the multidisciplinary team such as dieticians, stoma care nurses and nutrition nurses. Recently, a number of centres have introduced a dedicated ERAS nurse who provides information regarding ERAS pathways and the various stages during and after surgery. An important component of preoperative phase is the ingestion of carbohydrate-rich drink the night before and on the morning of surgery. A short period of fasting and carbohydrate loading both help in maintaining patients' nitrogen balance and reducing post-operative insulin resistance (Soop, et al. 2004; Svanfeldt, et al. 2007).

Oral mechanical bowel preparation should be avoided in patients undergoing elective bowel surgery. A single phosphate enema can be used on the days of surgery to clear the rectum in patients undergoing left-sided anastomosis. A Cochrane review suggested that low molecular weight heparin (LMWH) and graduated compression thromboembolic deterrent stockings (TEDs) are the most effective anti-thrombotic prophylaxis (Wille-Jorgensen, et al. 2003). A single dose of broad spectrum antibiotics reduces the risk of wound infection and should be administered prior to skin incision.

4.1.3 Peri-operative components of ERAS protocols

High inspired oxygen concentrations (80%) should be administered during anaesthesia and in the early post-operative period (for a minimum of six hours). Oxygen molecules are required for the production of free radicals, which play an important role in the defence mechanism against pathogens to reduce surgical site infection, and in the synthesis of collagen for wound healing and angiogenensis (Allen, et al. 1997; Hopf, et al. 1997; Qadan, et al. 2009). In addition, high concentration of oxygen in the tissues during the immediate post-operative period improves perfusion at the anastomotic site and may also be associated with a reduction in post-operative nausea and vomiting (PONV) (Greif, et al. 1999; Orhan-Sungur, et al. 2008).

The core temperature should be measured and monitored using an oesophageal probe. In patients undergoing prolonged surgery (i.e., more than one hour) warmed intravenous fluid should be administered (Lindwall, et al. 1998; Smith, et al. 1998).

Hypothermia (core temperature less than 36°C) causes tissue hypoxia due to peripheral vasoconstriction which increases the risk of coagulopathy, wound infections and cardiac complications (Frank, et al. 1997; Ozaki, et al. 1995; Schmied, et al. 1996). It is also linked to a change in immune response and an increase in catabolic response (Frank, et al. 1995). Prevention of hypothermia in the peri-operative phase has been shown to decrease blood loss, and cardiac and infective complications (Melling, et al. 2001; Wong, et al. 2007).

Goal directed intra-operative intravenous fluid administration has shown positive impact on early return of gut function and reduction in length of stay in hospital. Oesophageal Doppler or LiDCO plus™ and LiDCO rapid™ are minimally invasive methods used to measure the cardiac output and stroke volume. These devices enable the anaesthetist to tailor the fluid requirement (goal directed) according to changes in cardiac output per-operatively. Goal directed fluid therapy has been shown to result in early return of gastric motility, reduction in time to defecation and an improved tolerance to oral feed due to reduced gut oedema (Gan, et al. 2002; Lobo, et al. 2002; Nisanevich, et al. 2005) . Splanchnic hypoperfusion, which may remain unnoticed with traditional monitoring, results in delayed return of gut function. It may lead to bacterial translocation across the gut wall and sepsis (Mythen and Webb 1994). Similarly, an excessive amount of intravenous fluid during surgery may cause the development of gut oedema which may also result in the delay in return of gut function (Grocott, et al. 2005).

The concept of minimally invasive surgery is recommended which includes both open (small and appropriate incisions) as well as laparoscopic approach. In open approach, a transverse, limited midline, oblique or paramedian incision should be used whenever possible. Such small transverse or mini-laparotomy incisions may have positive impact on analgesic requirement, pulmonary complications, systemic inflammatory response and length of stay in hospital

(Nakagoe, et al. 2001; Nakagoe, et al. 2004; Takegami, et al. 2003; Werawatganon and Charuluxanun 2005). In ERAS protocol, routine use of nasogastric tubes and abdominal drains following GI surgery is not recommended. A Cochrane review (33 studies, 5240 patients) has suggested that there was an earlier return of gut function, reduction in pulmonary complications and an insignificant trend towards increased risk of wound infection in patients not having routine nasogastric tube. However, no difference in the rates of anastomotic dehiescence was demonstrated. Its use is also associated with pain and discomfort to patient and impedes post-operative mobility (Nelson, et al. 2007; Nelson, et al. 2005). Similarly, several randomised studies and meta-analyses have suggested that the routine use of drains does not confer any clinical advantage in the early detection of anastomotic leak or intra-abdominal collection (Jesus, et al. 2004; Karliczek, et al. 2006; Urbach, et al. 1999).

It is recommended that all patients undergoing open abdominal surgery should have high thoracic epidural analgesia. Patient should receive epidural analgesia for at least 12 hours to a maximum of 48 hours. Ideally weaning form epidural should start 12 hours after operation.

However, in laparoscopic colorectal surgery the benefits of epidural analgesia are not clear. It may be used depending upon the preference of the operating surgeon and anaesthetist. The epidural anaesthesia blocks sympathetic reflexes and afferent stimuli. This attenuates the post-operative stress and promotes early return of gut function which reduces incidence of PIO (Holte and Kehlet 2002; Marret, et al. 2007). It is important to note that epidural analgesia may cause hypotension due to vasodilatation which may have an adverse affect on the anastomosis. Early recognition of these patients and monitoring in the high dependency unit is therfore critical.

Recently, other modalities such as transversus abdominis plane (TAP) blocks and wound irrigation (PainBuster®) with local anaesthetic (0.2% ropivacaine®) have shown a reduction in use of opiates and improvement in patient mobilisation in the early post-operative period (Bamigboye and Hofmeyr 2009; Beaussier, et al. 2007).

4.1.4 Post-operative components of ERAS protocols

Opiates have a profound negative effect on the gut motility, consequently delaying return of gut function and prolonging the duration of POI. Regular use of Paracetamol and non-steroidal anti-inflammatory drugs (NSAIDS) is recommended unless contraindicated. NSAIDS help promote gut recovery by reducing local mucosal inflammation (Cali, et al. 2000). Prophylactic antiemetics should be prescribed to those patients receiving opiates.

It is emphasised that all patients be allowed oral fluid and diet soon after surgery. Intravenous fluid should be stopped as soon as the patient's oral intake is adequate. There is now evidence to support the view that early commencement of enteral feeding is beneficial and is safe to introduce within 24 hours of surgery (Andersen, et al. 2006; Lewis, et al. 2009). Similarly, early feeding facilitates gut motility and may help in the early return of gut function and reduce the ileus.

All patients should have an enforced and structured mobilisation plan during the post-operative period. A designated physiotherapist with a mobilisation plan tailored to the individual patient's need should work closely with the patient in order to achieve best outcome. Early mobilisation is paramount in preventing venous thromboembolism (VTE), respiratory complications and reduction in muscle strength (Schuster and Montie 2002). It is noteworthy that early post-operative ambulation plays a little role in preventing or resolving POI. However, it has proven benefits in preventing atelectasis, pneumonia and VTE (Carroll and Alavi 2009) which may cause secondary POI.

A clinical management pathway, based on ERAS protocols, is proposed below which would be useful for colorectal surgeons in day-to-day management of surgical patients (Figure- 3).

A typical pathway for management of patients after colorectal surgery - Based on multimodal optimisation

Preoperative Phase

Patient counselling and education (both written and verbal) Assessment by Anaesthetist and ERAS Nurse Optimisation of nutritional status (MUST scoring) and co-morbidities Stoma education and training (if required)	Preoperative assessment
Carbohydrate loading Clear fluids till 2 hours prior to surgery Bowel prep (if required) VTE prophylaxis No premedication	Day of admission

Peroperative Phase

Epidural analgesia Goal directed IV fluids (Use Oesophageal Doppler) No nasogastric tube or drains Prophylactic antibiotics Minimally invasive surgical approach (laparoscopic/ small / transverse incision)	In operating theatre

Postoperative Phase

Set of daily goals for postoperative care Start oral fluids and diet as soon as patient tolerates Regular paracetamol and NSAID if not contraindicated Continue high energy drinks Avoid regular Morphine and other opiates Daily review by physio and active and enforced mobilisation	In HDU/ward

Fig. 3. Clinical management pathway based on ERAS protocols

4.2 Laparoscopic approach

Introduction of laparoscopic approach has significant imapct on surgical practice, for both the surgeons and patients alike. It is known that the laparoscopic techniques cause less surgical stress and trauma, and the patients recover faster (Bauer and Boeckxstaens 2004; Kalff, et al. 1998). Laparoscopic surgery involves less bowel manipulation and inflicts reduced tissue trauma compared with open approach. Similarly, reduced inflammatory and catabolic responses in laparoscopic approach may also result in early recovery after operation. Therefore, the return of gut function is faster compared to open surgery. Effective postoperative analgesia may be obtained with simple analgesics and use of opiates can easily be avoided. Understandably, laparoscopic technique is considered to reduce severity and duration of ileus resulting in shorther length of stay in hospital (Leung, et al. 2004).

Laparoscopic technique has attracted ethusiasm and application by most surgical specialities and has become standard approach for a number of surgical procedures. Its wide spread popularity is based on the short term benefits. Randomised studies have demonstrated that laparoscopic approach reduces duration of POI after abdominal surgery (Basse, et al. 2003; Lacy, et al. 1995; Milsom, et al. 1998). Similarly, laparoscopic colorectal resections have been shown to cause less post-operative pain, and early return of organ function and discharge from hospital when compared with conventional open surgery (Reza, et al. 2006).

Whereas individual trials demostrate short term benefits of laparoscopic approach especially in early postoperative period (Guillou, et al. 2005; Murray, et al. 2006; Veldkamp, et al. 2005), a Cochrane review found no difference in long term outcomes compared with open approach (Kuhry, et al. 2008). However, it is important to consider that most of above evidence is collected from studies lacking ERAS programme of perioperative optimisation. Recently, two trials investigated impact of laparoscopic approach within ERAS application (Basse, et al. 2005; King, et al. 2006). Unfortunately, the results of these two trials are not consistent. Basse et al. failed to show any advantage of laparoscopic approach in colonic resections, while King et al suggested benefits of laparoscopic approach compared with open techniques. However, latter trial was not blinded which might have impacted on the results of the study. Nevertheless, it is established that laparoscopic surgery, in general, is associated with reduced post operative pain and inflammatory response. Consequently, it may play a role in reducing the incidence of POI (Story and Chamberlain 2009). More work is underway in this area and evidence is eagerly awaited.

4.3 Pharmacological therapies

There are a number of pharmacological therapies which are part of ERAS protocols. For instance, carbohydrate loading, use of NSAID and prophylactic anti-emetics, epidural and/or regional analgesia are integral part of ERAS pathways. These therapeutic modalities have been shown to have significant impact on early return of gut function (Kehlet and Wilmore 2008). Moreover, it is possible to avoid opiates which have a profound effect on gut motility and cause ileus.

A number of new pharmacological agents are under investigation at different levels. For example, Alvimopan, a selective Mu-opioid receptor antagonist which acts peripherally, has been shown to have positive effect on the ileus in phase III trail. It has been shown to have an association with early return of bowel function, reduced incidence of POI, and reduction in length of hospital stay (Ludwig, et al. 2010). Similarly, estimated hospital cost was reduced by $879 - $977 for patients who received alvimopan compared with placebo. Long-term safety, accurate indications and dosage are important issues which need addressing before its widespread use in future. However, it is unknown that if alvimopan is more cost effective than optimal use of laparoscopic approach and ERAS protocols, and further research is needed (Stewart and Waxman 2010).

Similarly, vagal stimulation by enteral administration of lipid-rich nutrition has shown early recovery of gut peristalsis (Lubbers, et al. 2010). Other agents such as peripheral opioid antagonist methylnaltrexone, motilin analogue atilmotin and Cisapride have been used with promising results (Livingston and Passaro 1990). Adrenergic blockers and parasympathetic agonists (e.g neostigmine) have also been investigated as potential options in treating POI. Unfortunately, these agents have serious side effects and hence not suitable for routine practice. Moreover, drugs such as Erythromycin and Metoclopramide have shown some favourable results in early gastric emptying, however, there is no quality data to support their routine use at a larger scale in daily practice (Sustic, et al. 2005; Yeo, et al. 1993). A recent review suggested that gum chewing in postoperative period is associated with reduction in POI, likely due to vagal stimulation of the gastrointestinal tract (Fitzgerald and Ahmed 2009).

The pharmacological management of POI is still evolving and has an important role in the management of POI. Further evidence is required to establish the summative effect of pharmacological therapies, laparoscopic surgery and ERAS pathways.

5. Conclusion

POI is a complex condition of multifactorial aetiology, most commonly seen following abdominal surgery. It causes significant frustration amongst health professionals and patients alike. It is one of the commonest causes of delay in patients' postoperative recovery and carries financial implications due to prolonged length of stay. It is estimated to cost $1.28 billion annually in United States (Senagore 2007).

In recent years, efforts have been made to address this issue albeit without any major progress. Nonetheless, our understanding of pathophysiology of ileus is better than before and a number of strategies to overcome the causative factors have been tried (Stewart and Waxman 2010; Story and Chamberlain 2009). Although such strategies help reduce the duration of ileus, they have limited role in preventing its onset (Lubawski and Saclarides 2008). Three major mechanisms - neurogenic, inflammatory and pharmacological - have been implicated in causing ileus (Augestad and Delaney 2010). The level of activation of these factors varies during a surgical procedure. Moreover, understanding of pharmacological mechanisms has opened new windows for research and interventions in this area.

Evidence has accumulated to suggest enhanced recovery after surgery protocol, laparoscopic approach, and pharmacological interventions all reduce the incidence of ileus. Figure 4 illustrates a suggested pathway for prevention and management of prolonged Ileus.

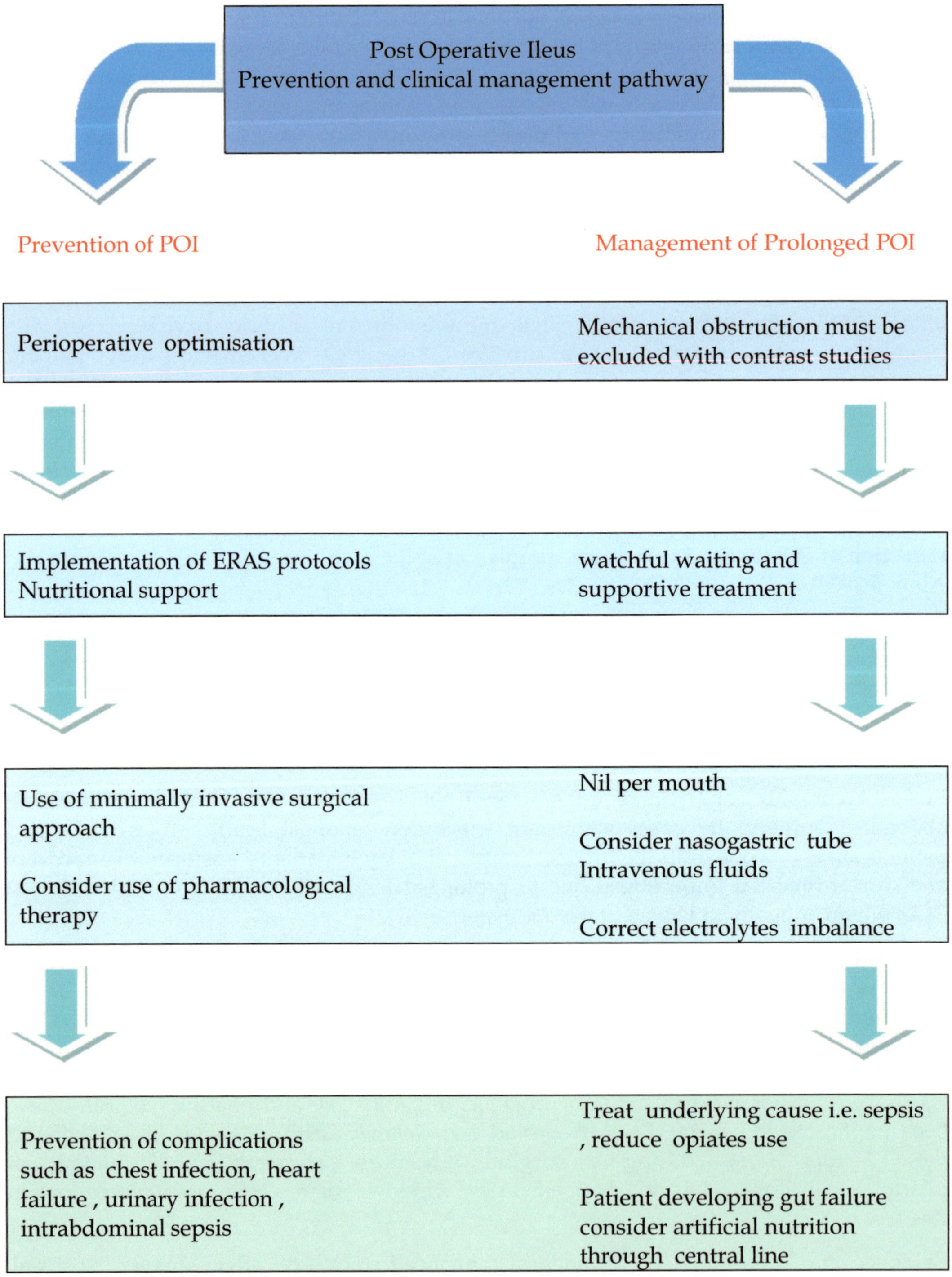

Fig. 4. Management pathway for Prolonged POI

Laparoscopic surgery produces better short term results compared with open approach (Guillou, et al. 2005; Hewett, et al. 2008). Short term morbidity, including incidence of ileus, is significantly low in patients treated with laparoscopic approach. It remains an area of significant reserach interest to investigate whether the combination of laparoscopic surgery and ERAS protocol will offer any further clinical benefit. The ongoing LAFA (Dutch) and EnRoL (UK) trials are desinged to answer above question when completed (Wind, et al. 2006a).

Of above, ERAS pathway was most extensively studied intervention over the last 15 years.The components of ERAS protocol are aimed at optimising patient care, reducing operative stress, and enhancing recovery after surgery by persevering normal physiology and early return of gastrointestinal function. Whereas POI has not been investigated as sole primary endpoint in studies comparing ERAS verusu conventional perioperative care, it has been studied as a part of morbidity rates in both as primary and secondary endpoints. There is now evidence that ERAS protocol of perioperative care is associated with significant reduction in incidence of POI, along with length of hospital stay, compared with conventional perioperative care.

Pharmacological interventions, as part of ERAS or outside ERAS, play key role in reduction of incidence of ileus. Such interventions with promising results include use of preoperative carbohydrate loading, NSAIDs, prophylactic anti-emetics, and epidural and/or regional analgesia. Avoidance of opiates and use of mu-opoid receptor antagonists are associated with early return of gut function.

The impact of ileus as an important health issue cannot be over emphasized:

"In patients who underwent colectomy surgery, postoperative ileus was associated with a 29% increase in hospital LOS and a 15% increase in hospitalization costs. Prevention of postoperative ileus could potentially yield benefits in reduction in hospital LOS and associated health care costs." (Lyer, et al. 2009)

POI is a challenging yet preventable event in surgical patients. It has a multifactorial pathophysiology that requires a multimodal approach in its management. Whereas there is no definitive treatment of ileus, strategies to prevent and manage ileus should be followed as discussed above. Essentially, prevention and management of POI centres on minimising perioperative stress and preserving normal physiological functions.

6. References

2004 A comparison of laparoscopically assisted and open colectomy for colon cancer. N Engl J Med 350(20):2050-9.

Ahmed, J., et al. 2010 Compliance with enhanced recovery programmes in elective colorectal surgery. Br J Surg 97(5):754-8.

Allen, D. B., et al. 1997 Wound hypoxia and acidosis limit neutrophil bacterial killing mechanisms. Arch Surg 132(9):991-6.

Andersen, H. K., S. J. Lewis, and S. Thomas 2006 Early enteral nutrition within 24h of colorectal surgery versus later commencement of feeding for postoperative complications. Cochrane Database Syst Rev (4):CD004080.

Asgeirsson, T., et al. 2010 Postoperative ileus: it costs more than you expect. J Am Coll Surg 210(2):228-31.

Augestad, K. M., and C. P. Delaney 2010 Postoperative ileus: impact of pharmacological treatment, laparoscopic surgery and enhanced recovery pathways. World J Gastroenterol 16(17):2067-74.

Bamigboye, A. A., and G. J. Hofmeyr 2009 Local anaesthetic wound infiltration and abdominal nerves block during caesarean section for postoperative pain relief. Cochrane Database Syst Rev (3):CD006954.

Barquist, E., et al. 1996 Neuronal pathways involved in abdominal surgery-induced gastric ileus in rats. Am J Physiol 270(4 Pt 2):R888-94.

Basse, L., et al. 2005 Functional recovery after open versus laparoscopic colonic resection: a randomized, blinded study. Ann Surg 241(3):416-23.

— 2003 Gastrointestinal transit after laparoscopic versus open colonic resection. Surg Endosc 17(12):1919-22.

Bauer, A. J., and G. E. Boeckxstaens 2004 Mechanisms of postoperative ileus. Neurogastroenterol Motil 16 Suppl 2:54-60.

Bauer, A. J., M. G. Sarr, and J. H. Szurszewski 1991 Opioids inhibit neuromuscular transmission in circular muscle of human and baboon jejunum. Gastroenterology 101(4):970-6.

Bauer AJ, Szurszewski JH. 1991 Effect of opioid peptides on circular muscle of canine duodenum j Physiol 434:409- 422.

Beaussier, M., et al. 2007 Continuous preperitoneal infusion of ropivacaine provides effective analgesia and accelerates recovery after colorectal surgery: a randomized, double-blind, placebo-controlled study. Anesthesiology 107(3):461-8.

Boeckxstaens, G. E., and W. J. de Jonge 2009 Neuroimmune mechanisms in postoperative ileus. Gut 58(9):1300-11.

Boeckxstaens, G. E., et al. 1999 Activation of an adrenergic and vagally-mediated NANC pathway in surgery-induced fundic relaxation in the rat. Neurogastroenterol Motil 11(6):467-74.

— 2000 Evidence for VIP(1)/PACAP receptors in the afferent pathway mediating surgery-induced fundic relaxation in the rat. Br J Pharmacol 131(4):705-10.

Bonaz, B., and Y. Tache 1997 Corticotropin-releasing factor and systemic capsaicin-sensitive afferents are involved in abdominal surgery-induced Fos expression in the paraventricular nucleus of the hypothalamus. Brain Res 748(1-2):12-20.

Cali, R. L., et al. 2000 Effect of Morphine and incision length on bowel function after colectomy. Dis Colon Rectum 43(2):163-8.

Carroll, J., and K. Alavi 2009 Pathogenesis and management of postoperative ileus. Clin Colon Rectal Surg 22(1):47-50.

Cicalese, L., et al. 1996 Pyruvate prevents mucosal reperfusion injury, oxygen free-radical production, and neutrophil infiltration after rat small bowel preservation and transplantation. Transplant Proc 28(5):2611.

Cochrane, J. P., et al. 1981 Arginine vasopressin release following surgical operations. Br J Surg 68(3):209-13.

de Jonge, W. J., et al. 2003 Postoperative ileus is maintained by intestinal immune infiltrates that activate inhibitory neural pathways in mice. Gastroenterology 125(4):1137-47.

De Winter, B. Y., et al. 1997 Effect of adrenergic and nitrergic blockade on experimental ileus in rats. Br J Pharmacol 120(3):464-8.

— 1998 Role of VIP1/PACAP receptors in postoperative ileus in rats. Br J Pharmacol 124(6):1181-6.

Delaney C, Kehlet H, Senagore A, et al 2006 Postoperative ileus: profiles, risk factors, and definitions—a framework for optimizing surgical outcomes in patients undergoing major abdominal colorectal surgery. Clinical consensus update in general surgery.:26.

Dubois, A., D. P. Henry, and I. J. Kopin 1975 Plasma catecholamines and postoperative gastric emptying and small intestinal propulsion in the rat. Gastroenterology 68(3):466-9.

Faussone-Pellegrini, M. S., D. Pantalone, and C. Cortesini 1990 Smooth muscle cells, interstitial cells of Cajal and myenteric plexus interrelationships in the human colon. Acta Anat (Basel) 139(1):31-44.

Finney, J. M. 1906 IV. Postoperative Ileus. Ann Surg 43(6):870-904.

Fitzgerald, J. E., and I. Ahmed 2009 Systematic review and meta-analysis of chewing-gum therapy in the reduction of postoperative paralytic ileus following gastrointestinal surgery. World J Surg 33(12):2557-66.

Frank, S. M., et al. 1997 Perioperative maintenance of normothermia reduces the incidence of morbid cardiac events. A randomized clinical trial. JAMA 277(14):1127-34.

— 1995 The catecholamine, cortisol, and hemodynamic responses to mild perioperative hypothermia. A randomized clinical trial. Anesthesiology 82(1):83-93.

Gan, T. J., et al. 2002 Goal-directed intraoperative fluid administration reduces length of hospital stay after major surgery. Anesthesiology 97(4):820-6.

Greif, R., et al. 1999 Supplemental oxygen reduces the incidence of postoperative nausea and vomiting. Anesthesiology 91(5):1246-52.

Grocott, M. P., M. G. Mythen, and T. J. Gan 2005 Perioperative fluid management and clinical outcomes in adults. Anesth Analg 100(4):1093-106.

Gue, M., et al. 1989 Stimulation of kappa opiate receptors in intestinal wall affects stress-induced increase of plasma cortisol in dogs. Brain Res 502(1):143-8.

Guillou, P. J., et al. 2005 Short-term endpoints of conventional versus laparoscopic-assisted surgery in patients with colorectal cancer (MRC CLASICC trial): multicentre, randomised controlled trial. Lancet 365(9472):1718-26.

Hewett, P. J., et al. 2008 Short-term outcomes of the Australasian randomized clinical study comparing laparoscopic and conventional open surgical treatments for colon cancer: the ALCCaS trial. Ann Surg 248(5):728-38.

Holte, K., and H. Kehlet 2000 Postoperative ileus: a preventable event. Br J Surg 87(11):1480-93.

— 2002 Epidural anaesthesia and analgesia - effects on surgical stress responses and implications for postoperative nutrition. Clin Nutr 21(3):199-206.

Hopf, H. W., et al. 1997 Wound tissue oxygen tension predicts the risk of wound infection in surgical patients. Arch Surg 132(9):997-1004; discussion 1005.

Iyer, S., W. B. Saunders, and S. Stemkowski 2009. Economic burden of postoperative ileus associated with colectomy in the United States. J Manag Care Pharm 15(6):485-94.

Jesus, E. C., et al. 2004 Prophylactic anastomotic drainage for colorectal surgery. Cochrane Database Syst Rev (4):CD002100.

Kagan, B. L., T. Ganz, and R. I. Lehrer 1994 Defensins: a family of antimicrobial and cytotoxic peptides. Toxicology 87(1-3):131-49.

Kalff, J. C., et al. 1999 Surgically induced leukocytic infiltrates within the rat intestinal muscularis mediate postoperative ileus. Gastroenterology 117(2):378-87.

— 1998 Surgical manipulation of the gut elicits an intestinal muscularis inflammatory response resulting in postsurgical ileus. Ann Surg 228(5):652-63.

Kalff, J. C., Schraut WH, Billiar TR, Simmons RL, Baur AJ, 1999 Roles of inducible nitric oxide synthase in postoperative intestinal smooth muscle dysfunction in rodents. . Gastroenterology 188:316-27.

Karliczek, A., et al. 2006 Drainage or nondrainage in elective colorectal anastomosis: a systematic review and meta-analysis. Colorectal Dis 8(4):259-65.

Kehlet, H., and D. W. Wilmore 2008 Evidence-based surgical care and the evolution of fast-track surgery. Ann Surg 248(2):189-98.

Khoo, C. K., et al. 2007 A prospective randomized controlled trial of multimodal perioperative management protocol in patients undergoing elective colorectal resection for cancer. Ann Surg 245(6):867-72.

King, P. M., et al. 2006 Randomized clinical trial comparing laparoscopic and open surgery for colorectal cancer within an enhanced recovery programme. Br J Surg 93(3):300-8.

Kubes, P., and S. Kanwar 1994 Histamine induces leukocyte rolling in post-capillary venules. A P-selectin-mediated event. J Immunol 152(7):3570-7.

Kuhry, E., et al. 2008 Long-term results of laparoscopic colorectal cancer resection. Cochrane Database Syst Rev (2):CD003432.

Kurz, A., and D. I. Sessler 2003 Opioid-induced bowel dysfunction: pathophysiology and potential new therapies. Drugs 63(7):649-71.

Lacy, A. M., et al. 1995 Short-term outcome analysis of a randomized study comparing laparoscopic vs open colectomy for colon cancer. Surg Endosc 9(10):1101-5.

Leung, K. L., et al. 2004 Laparoscopic resection of rectosigmoid carcinoma: prospective randomised trial. Lancet 363(9416):1187-92.

Lewis, S. J., H. K. Andersen, and S. Thomas 2009 Early enteral nutrition within 24 h of intestinal surgery versus later commencement of feeding: a systematic review and meta-analysis. J Gastrointest Surg 13(3):569-75.

Lindwall, R., et al. 1998 Forced air warming and intraoperative hypothermia. Eur J Surg 164(1):13-6.

Livingston, E. H., and E. P. Passaro, Jr. 1990 Postoperative ileus. Dig Dis Sci 35(1):121-32.

Lobo, D. N., et al. 2002 Effect of salt and water balance on recovery of gastrointestinal function after elective colonic resection: a randomised controlled trial. Lancet 359(9320):1812-8.

Lubawski, J., and T. Saclarides 2008 Postoperative ileus: strategies for reduction. Ther Clin Risk Manag 4(5):913-7.

Lubbers, T., W. Buurman, and M. Luyer 2010 Controlling postoperative ileus by vagal activation. World J Gastroenterol 16(14):1683-7.

Luckey, A., E. Livingston, and Y. Tache 2003 Mechanisms and treatment of postoperative ileus. Arch Surg 138(2):206-14.

Ludwig, K., et al. 2010 Alvimopan for the management of postoperative ileus after bowel resection: characterization of clinical benefit by pooled responder analysis. World J Surg 34(9):2185-90.

Marret, E., C. Remy, and F. Bonnet 2007 Meta-analysis of epidural analgesia versus parenteral opioid analgesia after colorectal surgery. Br J Surg 94(6):665-73.

Mattei, P., and J. L. Rombeau 2006 Review of the pathophysiology and management of postoperative ileus. World J Surg 30(8):1382-91.

Melling, A. C., et al. 2001 Effects of preoperative warming on the incidence of wound infection after clean surgery: a randomised controlled trial. Lancet 358(9285):876-80.

Miedema, B. W., and J. O. Johnson 2003 Methods for decreasing postoperative gut dysmotility. Lancet Oncol 4(6):365-72.

Mikkelsen, H. B. 1995 Macrophages in the external muscle layers of mammalian intestines. Histol Histopathol 10(3):719-36.

Milsom, J. W., et al. 1998 A prospective, randomized trial comparing laparoscopic versus conventional techniques in colorectal cancer surgery: a preliminary report. J Am Coll Surg 187(1):46-54; discussion 54-5.

Mitchell, A., and J. Collin 1985 Vasopressin effects on the small intestine: a possible factor in paralytic ileus? Br J Surg 72(6):462-5.

Murray, A., et al. 2006 Clinical effectiveness and cost-effectiveness of laparoscopic surgery for colorectal cancer: systematic reviews and economic evaluation. Health Technol Assess 10(45):1-141, iii-iv.

Mythen, M. G., and A. R. Webb 1994 The role of gut mucosal hypoperfusion in the pathogenesis of post-operative organ dysfunction. Intensive Care Med 20(3):203-9.

Nakagoe, T., et al. 2001 Use of minilaparotomy in the treatment of colonic cancer. Br J Surg 88(6):831-6.

— 2004 Minilaparotomy approach for the resection of laterally spreading tumors of the colon. Surg Today 34(9):737-41.

Nelson, R., S. Edwards, and B. Tse 2007 Prophylactic nasogastric decompression after abdominal surgery. Cochrane Database Syst Rev (3):CD004929.

Nelson, R., B. Tse, and S. Edwards 2005 Systematic review of prophylactic nasogastric decompression after abdominal operations. Br J Surg 92(6):673-80.

Nisanevich, V., et al. 2005 Effect of intraoperative fluid management on outcome after intraabdominal surgery. Anesthesiology 103(1):25-32.

Orhan-Sungur, M., et al. 2008 Does supplemental oxygen reduce postoperative nausea and vomiting? A meta-analysis of randomized controlled trials. Anesth Analg 106(6):1733-8.

Ozaki, M., et al. 1995 Nitrous oxide decreases the threshold for vasoconstriction less than sevoflurane or isoflurane. Anesth Analg 80(6):1212-6.

Parvizi, J., et al. 2008 Postoperative ileus after total joint arthroplasty. J Arthroplasty 23(3):360-5.

Prasad, M., and J. B. Matthews 1999 Deflating postoperative ileus. Gastroenterology 117(2):489-92.

Qadan, M., et al. 2009 Perioperative supplemental oxygen therapy and surgical site infection: a meta-analysis of randomized controlled trials. Arch Surg 144(4):359-66; discussion 366-7.

Reissman, P., F. Agachan, and S. D. Wexner 1996 Outcome of laparoscopic colorectal surgery in older patients. Am Surg 62(12):1060-3.

Reza, M. M., et al. 2006 Systematic review of laparoscopic versus open surgery for colorectal cancer. Br J Surg 93(8):921-8.

Schmied, H., et al. 1996 Mild hypothermia increases blood loss and transfusion requirements during total hip arthroplasty. Lancet 347(8997):289-92.

Schuster, T. G., and J. E. Montie 2002 Postoperative ileus after abdominal surgery. Urology 59(4):465-71.

Schwarz, N. T., et al. 2001 Prostanoid production via COX-2 as a causative mechanism of rodent postoperative ileus. Gastroenterology 121(6):1354-71.

Senagore, A. J. 2007 Pathogenesis and clinical and economic consequences of postoperative ileus. Am J Health Syst Pharm 64(20 Suppl 13):S3-7.

Smith, C. E., et al. 1998 Warming intravenous fluids reduces perioperative hypothermia in women undergoing ambulatory gynecological surgery. Anesth Analg 87(1):37-41.

Smith, J., K. A. Kelly, and R. M. Weinshilboum 1977 Pathophysiology of postoperative ileus. Arch Surg 112(2):203-9.

Soop, M., et al. 2004 Preoperative oral carbohydrate treatment attenuates endogenous glucose release 3 days after surgery. Clin Nutr 23(4):733-41.

Stewart, D., and K. Waxman
2010 Management of postoperative ileus. Dis Mon 56(4):204-14.

Story, S. K., and R. S. Chamberlain. 2009 A comprehensive review of evidence-based strategies to prevent and treat postoperative ileus. Dig Surg 26(4):265-75.

Sustic, A., et al.2005 Metoclopramide improves gastric but not gallbladder emptying in cardiac surgery patients with early intragastric enteral feeding: randomized controlled trial. Croat Med J 46(2):239-44.

Svanfeldt, M., et al. 2007 Randomized clinical trial of the effect of preoperative oral carbohydrate treatment on postoperative whole-body protein and glucose kinetics. Br J Surg 94(11):1342-50.

Tache, Y., et al. 1993 Role of CRF in stress-related alterations of gastric and colonic motor function. Ann N Y Acad Sci 697:233-43.

Takegami, K., et al. 2003 Minilaparotomy approach to colon cancer. Surg Today 33(6):414-20.

Urbach, D. R., E. D. Kennedy, and M. M. Cohen 1999 Colon and rectal anastomoses do not require routine drainage: a systematic review and meta-analysis. Ann Surg 229(2):174-80.

Varadhan, K. K., et al. 2010 The enhanced recovery after surgery (ERAS) pathway for patients undergoing major elective open colorectal surgery: a meta-analysis of randomized controlled trials. Clin Nutr 29(4):434-40.

Veldkamp, R., et al. 2005 Laparoscopic surgery versus open surgery for colon cancer: short-term outcomes of a randomised trial. Lancet Oncol 6(7):477-84.

Weiskopf, R. B., et al. 1987 Effects of fentanyl on vasopressin secretion in human subjects. J Pharmacol Exp Ther 242(3):970-3.

Werawatganon, T., and S. Charuluxanun 2005 Patient controlled intravenous opioid analgesia versus continuous epidural analgesia for pain after intra-abdominal surgery. Cochrane Database Syst Rev (1):CD004088.

Wershil, B. K., et al. 1996 Mast cell-dependent neutrophil and mononuclear cell recruitment in immunoglobulin E-induced gastric reactions in mice. Gastroenterology 110(5):1482-90.

Wille-Jorgensen, P., et al. 2003 Heparins and mechanical methods for thromboprophylaxis in colorectal surgery. Cochrane Database Syst Rev (4):CD001217.

Wind, J., et al. 2006a Perioperative strategy in colonic surgery; LAparoscopy and/or FAst track multimodal management versus standard care (LAFA trial). BMC Surg 6:16.

— 2006b Systematic review of enhanced recovery programmes in colonic surgery. Br J Surg 93(7):800-9.

Wong, P. F., et al. 2007 Randomized clinical trial of perioperative systemic warming in major elective abdominal surgery. Br J Surg 94(4):421-6.

Wood, J. D. 2008 Enteric nervous system: reflexes, pattern generators and motility. Curr Opin Gastroenterol 24(2):149-58.

Yeo, C. J., et al. 1993 Erythromycin accelerates gastric emptying after pancreaticoduodenectomy. A prospective, randomized, placebo-controlled trial. Ann Surg 218(3): 229-37; discussion 237-8.

Part 2

Laparoscopic Colorectal Surgery

3

Laparoscopic Surgery for Rectal Cancer: Approaches, Challenges and Outcome

Emad H. Aly
Aberdeen Royal Infirmary, Scotland
United Kingdom

1. Introduction

Jacobs et al (1991) reported the first series of laparoscopic colonic resections in 20 patients. It took over a decade of debate and controversy to establish that laparoscopic colon surgery for cancer, when compared with open surgery, is associated with better short term outcomes while maintaining at least equivalent long-term outcomes (Lee, 2009). These improved short term outcomes include reduced postoperative pain, short hospital stay, decreased intra-operative blood loss, quicker return of gut function and faster return to normal activities (Lacey et al., 2002; Veldkamp et al. ; 2005, Guillou et al., 2005). However, the debate around laparoscopic rectal surgery is far from over.

Oncologic outcomes of rectal cancer patients have been shown to depend on the skills and techniques of the operating surgeon (Heald et al., 1998). It took the surgical community several years to accept and adopt the current modern concepts of rectal cancer surgery which involves the standardisation of surgical resection with total mesorectal excision (Heald et al; 1986) and adequate circumferential resection margin (Quirke et al., 1988). It seems that the surgical community has yet to go through another phase of development in the surgical management of rectal cancer to address the concerns whether the technical challenges of laparoscopy may further add to the complexity of the surgical technique that may result in variability in outcomes (Lee, 2009).

Even though there are several studies on the outcomes of laparoscopic rectal surgery, there is limited level 1 evidence in surgical literature (Kang et al., 2010). Safety and benefits associated with laparoscopic colon cancer surgery have been demonstrated in many prospective randomized trials. However the same benefits have not yet been clearly confirmed for laparoscopic rectal cancer surgery (Lee, 2009). The debate around laparoscopic rectal surgery has become even more complex with the slow, but steady, increase of the practice of robotic rectal surgery. To be universally accepted, minimally invasive approaches to rectal cancer need to demonstrate at least equivalent onlcologic & safety results to open surgery combined with evidence of improved short term outcomes. In addition, minimally invasive approach should be cost-effective (Champagne et al., 2007).

2. Conventional laparoscopic rectal surgery

2.1 Pros and cons of conventional laparoscopic rectal surgery

Laparoscopic surgery provides unique, unobstructed views of the rectal dissection not only for the operating surgeon but also to the entire surgical team. Magnification of the surgical field allows more precise dissection. The pneumoperitoneum assists in opening up the planes for mobilization of the mesorectum (Lee, 2009). Also, blood loss is minimised as meticulous haemostasis is essential to preserve the laparoscopic view. (Cecil et al., 2006).

However, there are many well documented limitations to conventional laparoscopic rectal surgery. These include tremor, assistant dependant unstable two-dimensional view, inability to perform high-precision suturing, poor ergonomics and fixed tips as well as limited dexitry of surgical instruments (Delaney et al., 2003; Choi et al., 2009; Abodeely et al, 2010). These limitations are particularly relevant for rectal cancer surgery. As the surgeon operates into the confines of the pelvis the dissection becomes more difficult due to a combination of factors. Retraction of the rectum may prove difficult as one approaches the retrorectal and Denovillier's fascias. Crowding and clashing of instruments can result in a poor view and an experienced assistant is essential. Diathermy or vapour fumes from energy sources in the confined spaces of the pelvis often results in fogging of the camera scope that could slow progress of the procedure (Cecil et al., 2006).

2.2 Challenges in conventional laparoscopic rectal surgery

There are many technical challenges that are associated with laparoscopic rectal cancer surgery. One of the main technical challenges is obtaining adequate exposure, tissue tension & retraction of the rectum by the currently available conventional laparoscopic instruments. In the absence of tactile feedback during laparoscopic surgery, intra-operative localisation of the tumour represents another challenge. Lesions during laparoscopic colon surgery are easily identifiable with or without tattoo marks. However, this is not easily possible with rectal cancers without tactile feedback. It is often difficult to determine the extent of distal rectal dissection that is needed to grantee adequate tumour clearance and to be sure that the stapler is applied at the appropriate level distal to the tumour (Lee, 2009).

There are well known limitations in the currently available laparoscopic distal rectal stapling devices. Most of the current laparoscopic staplers can only reticulate to a maximum of 65 degrees which makes horizontal division of the rectum difficult. For this reason, multiple firings are often required to complete distal rectal transection (Cecil et al., 2006). Division of the rectum in the presence of very low anterior and bulky lesions is particularly challenging (Champagne et al., 2011). Laparoscopic division of the distal rectum is not always technically feasible because of the limited angulation of the stapling device and the physical limitations of working in the bony confines of the pelvis. A virtual simulation demonstrated that the current design of staplers has to go through the iliac bone in order to achieve a 90° angle at the level of levator ani (Brannigan et al., 2006). Some surgeons overcome by this by the use of a conventional stapler through a small suprapubic incision (Shalli et al., 2009).

Identifying the correct surgical plane anterior to Denonvillier's fascia during conventional laparoscopic rectal surgery, adequate radial margin and maintaining meticulous haemostasis are essential for high quality rectal cancer surgery. This can be challenging as without adequate retraction and tissue tension, surgical planes can be more ambiguous. Any bleeding will further obscure the appropriate anatomy (Champagne et al., 2011).

2.3 Outcomes of conventional laparoscopic rectal surgery

2.3.1 Evidence from early randomised controlled trials

The MRC CLASICC (**C**onventional vs. **L**aparoscopic- **A**ssisted **S**urgery in **C**olorectal **C**ancer) Trial was done between 1996 and 2002 in 27 UK centres. It randomised 794 patients with colon and rectal cancer into laparoscopic resection (n = 526) open resection (n = 268) with a ratio of 2:1. The CLASICC trial was the first RCT to include patients with rectal cancer. The study reported a 29% conversion rate. Patients who had conversion ended up with increased complication rates. Also, there was higher incidence of positive circumferential resection margin after laparoscopic anterior resection but this did not reach statistical significance. There was no difference in hospital mortality or quality of life at 2 weeks and 3 months postoperatively (Guillou et al., 2005).

A subset of 148 patients in the CLASICC trial was analyzed with regard to sexual and urinary function with the help of validated questionnaires. The perceived change in the overall level of sexual function was considerably higher in the laparoscopic group compared with the conventional group (41 vs 23%). These differences in sexual function reflected a clear trend, but were not significant at the 5% level.

Multivariate analysis revealed that conversion to open surgery was significantly correlated with postoperative male sexual dysfunction. In this study morbidity was an obvious issue in rectal surgery. Therefore, the authors concluded: *'laparoscopic resection for colon cancer is as effective as open surgery. However, impaired short-term outcomes after laparoscopic resection for rectal cancer do not yet justify its routine use. '* (Guillou et al., 2005).

2.3.2 Challenges in rectal surgery as identified from the clasicc trial

The outcomes of the MRC CLASICC trial should be interpreted with caution as in the study design, which was based on the best available data at that time (Simons et al., 1995), the surgeons' learning curve was set at 20 laparoscopic resections. Clearly this was an underestimation of the learning curve especially for rectal surgery (Leung et al., 2004; Good et al., 2011). This could explain the increased complication rate for laparoscopic rectal resections in the study and the authors' conclusion that laparoscopic rectal surgery was associated with increased morbidity. The reduction in the conversion rates for every year of the study is an indication that the learning curve was operative during the trial (Guillou et al, 2005). More recent studies set the learning curve at 55 cases for right-sided and 62 for left-sided laparoscopic colonic resections to achieve proficiency (Tekkis et al., 2005). However, there is little data on the numbers required to achieve proficiency in laparoscopic rectal cancer surgery (Good et al., 2011).

Despite the limitations of the MRC CLASICC trial, it helped to highlight the challenges of laparoscopic rectal surgery when compared to laparoscopic colon surgery. These findings were confirmed & debated in other publications (Quah et al., 2002; Scheidbach et al., 2002; Cecil et al., 2006). It became evident that laparoscopic rectal surgery has a longer learning curve & higher conversion rate, increased circumferential margin involvement as well as poorer outcome of urinary and sexual function especially in men (Quah et al., 2002; Bretagnol et al., 2005).

Increased anastomotic leak rate was another challenge that was identified in laparoscopic rectal surgery. Multiple firings are often required to complete distal rectal transection as the current laparoscopic staplers can only reticulate to a maximum of 65 degrees and therefore horizontal division of the rectum difficult. This is even more challenging for low-lying lesions and may contribute to increased anastomotic leakage. There is a documented positive relationship between the number of linear endostapler firings and anastomotic leak rate (Ito et al., 2008; Kim et al., 2009). Reported leak rate of 17% if the anastomosis were located less than 12 cm from the anal verge and as high as 25% in those patients who were not diverted following laparoscopic rectal surgery (Morino et al., 2003). These leak rates are higher than those reported after open rectal resection (4–11%) (Enker et al., 1995; Heald et al. 1998). Refinements in the laparoscopic stapling devices may help addressing this problem in the future.

2.3.3 Evidence from more recent publications

More recent publications show much lower rate of circumferential resection margin (CRM) involvement following conventional laparoscopic rectal surgery between 2. 14%-4% (Ng K. H. et al., 2009; Lujan et al., 2009; Ng SS et al., 2009). On the other hand, anastomotic leak rate remains high for most of the studies in the range of 9 to 17% compared to 5% for open surgery (Champagne et al., 2007). However, some authors report anastomotic leak rate after conventional laparoscopic rectal surgery as low as 3. 8% (Good et al., 2011).

2.3.4 Evidence from meta-analysis and cochrane reviews

The CRM involvement was evaluated in a meta-analysis of 10 trials reported a mean positive radial margin of 5% for laparoscopic resections compared with 8% for open resections. However, this was not statistically significant. The distal margin positivity rates were also not different between laparoscopic and open rectal surgery (Anderson et al., 2008). However, it should be noted that a clear distal margin can be of an issue in laparoscopic resections of the lower third of the rectum, especially in male patients (Laurent et al., 2007).

A meta-analysis for 20 studies published between 1993 and 2004 looking at laparoscopic versus open surgery for rectal cancer showed that there was no significant difference in circumferential margin positivity or number of lymph nodes harvested. This confirmed that laparoscopic and open surgery were comparable in terms of their adequacy of oncological clearance (Aziz et al., 2006). Despite the known limitations of meta-analysis of nonrandomized data, the authors' conclusions are particularly useful because of the limited number of randomized data available for laparoscopic rectal cancer surgery (Champagne et al., 2007).

A Cochran systematic review for 48 studies comparing laparoscopic and open resection for rectal cancer concluded that laparoscopic TME surgery had clinically measurable short-term advantages in patients with primary resectable rectal cancer (Breukink et al., 2006).

2.3.5 Outcomes of conventional laparoscopic resection of extra-peritoneal rectal cancer in recent studies

The ongoing debate as to the exact length of the rectum makes it difficult to accurately assess the results of the various studies reporting the outcomes of laparoscopic rectal surgery. Despite these apparent discrepancies there is an agreement that rectal cancer consists of extra-peritoneal and intra-peritoneal lesions and those tumours at or below the peritoneal reflection ideally should be grouped together (Champagne et al., 2011) when discussing laparoscopic rectal cancer outcomes because those lesions represent the real challenge for conventional laparoscopic rectal surgery. There is only limited number of studies that specifically address short and long term outcomes of conventional laparoscopic resection of these lesions.

Short-term Outcomes:

***COREAN Trial** (Comparison of **O**pen versus laparoscopic surgery for mid and low **RE**ctal cancer **A**fter **N**eoadjuvant chemoradiotherapy)*

This randomised study by Kang et al. (2010) aimed to evaluate the safety and short-term efficacy of laparoscopic surgery for rectal cancer after preoperative chemoradiotherapy. It was done between 2006-2009 in three tertiary referral centres by teams who have extensive experience in open and laparoscopic rectal surgery. Short-term outcomes assessed were involvement of the circumferential resection margin, macroscopic quality of the total mesorectal excision specimen, number of harvested lymph nodes, recovery of bowel function, perioperative morbidity, postoperative pain, and quality of life. Patients were followed up to assess the 3-year disease-free survival.

Conversion rate was 1. 2%. Laparoscopic group had a longer operating time but less post-operative pain, decreased blood loss and better physical functioning score. There was no difference between the two groups in the involvement of the circumferential resection margin, macroscopic quality of the total mesorectal excision specimen, number of harvested lymph nodes, and peri-operative morbidity did not differ between the two groups. The authors concluded that *'Laparoscopic surgery after preoperative chemoradiotherapy for mid or low rectal cancer is safe and has short-term benefits compared with open surgery; the quality of oncological resection was equivalent'* (Kang et al., 2010).

Even though the COREAN study showed no statistical difference in the anastomotic leak rate between the open and laparoscopic groups, other recent studies have highlighted that laparoscopic resection of extraperitoneal rectal cancer is associated with increased anastomotic leak rate when compared to open surgery. Reported anastomotic leak rate following conventional laparoscopic low anterior resection is 9% (Morino et al., 2003; zhu et al., 2010) and up to 43% for an ultralow anterior resection (Choi et al., 2010).

Long-term Outcomes:

There is limited number of studies looking at the long-term prognosis following laparoscopic surgical resection of middle and lower rectal cancers. The long term outcomes in this subgroup of patients remain unclear because they are affected by anatomical factors as well as the complexity of the surgical procedures. Li et al. (2011) reported the outcome of 236 patients (laparoscopic, n = 113; open, n = 123) who underwent curative resection for middle and lower rectal cancer from 2000 to 2005. Surgery was performed by the same surgical team with extensive experience in laparoscopic and open procedures. The mean follow-up time of all patients was 74. 8 months. There was no statistical differences in local recurrence, distant recurrence or the 5-year overall survival rates between the laparoscopic and open groups. The authors concluded that *'laparoscopic and open surgery for middle and lower rectal cancer offer similar long-term outcomes. The continued use of laparoscopic surgery in these patients can be supported'*.

3. Hybrid and hand-assisted laparoscopic rectal surgery

In an attempt to avoid compromising oncologic rectal dissection but at the same time maintain the benefits of laparoscopic surgery some have studies reported the use of hybrid procedures in which colonic portion of the surgery is completed by the laparoscopic approach but rectal dissection is completed through a limited low midline or Pfannenstiel incision (Vithiananthan et al., 2001; Shalli et al., 2009).

Similarly, hand-assisted laparoscopic techniques have been used for rectal cancer surgery. Rectal exposure and dissection can be either performed directly through the hand assisted port incision using the open approach following laparoscopic mobilisation of the colon or laparoscopically with manual assistance. The latter technique uses the benefits of the unmatched laparoscopic view and at the same time allow the completion of oncologically similar dissection under tension as in open surgery (Lee et al., 2007).

Hybrid laparoscopic surgery allows the preservation of tactile sensation; optimal traction and exposure of the surgical planes and at the same time helps tumour localization which is a well known challenge in purely laparoscopic approach. Outcomes with this technique have been reported to be favourable and it certainly has some advantages but many surgeons feel that it is not 'totally' laparoscopic rectal surgery and it should not be included in trials or case series for laparoscopic rectal resection. However, the published literature highlights its role and it is suggested that if this procedure continues to demonstrate favourable outcomes and has a shorter learning curve it may require its own procedure code in the future (Champagne et al., 2011).

4. Robotic assisted rectal surgery

The inherent limitations of conventional laparoscopic surgery; which include tremor, unstable two-dimensional view, and limited degree of freedom of the instruments, are particularly significant in patients undergoing rectal cancer surgery with total mesorectal excision (Ballantyne, 2002). Robotic surgery has the potential to address some of these limitations and the potential to offer technical abilities greater than those offered by open or conventional laparoscopic surgery. Robotic colorectal surgery was first reported in by Ballantyne et al. in 2001. The concept of robotic total mesorectal excision for rectal cancer was first reported by Pigazzi et al. in 2006.

4.1 Potential advantages of robotic surgery

Robotic systems can address many of the inherent limitations of conventional laparoscopic surgery. These include the fulcrum effect, poor depth perception, limited range of motion as wells as instrument tremor (Maeso et al., 2010). The use of robotic systems in rectal cancer surgery has the potential to offer accurate dissection in the avascular 'holly' plane of the rectum without injury to the integrity of the mesorectum or autonomic pelvic nerves in the narrow pelvic cavity. Ultralow rectal dissection could be more easily performed by using precise movements of robotic arms (Kim & Kang, 2010).

Robotic system offers a camera system that is controlled by the operating surgeon combined with three dimensional ten-fold magnification vision thus allowing a perfectly still visibility of the operative field. (Ballantyne & Moll, 2003; Lanfranco et al., 2004; Baik, 2008). One of the main advantages of the use of robotic system in rectal surgery is that it gives the surgeon equal access to both right and left pelvis as if standing above the head of the patient (Hellan et al., 2007). The tips of the instruments of a robotic arm have an endowrist which has functions of seven degrees of freedom, one hundred and eighty degrees articulation and five hundred and forty degrees rotation (Baik, 2008). Also the availability of multi-articulated instruments allows for a range of angles to approach the rectum thus allowing sharp dissection around the rectum and mesorectum. The robotic handles transfer the hand movements of the surgeon to the tip of the instruments offering a comfortable, ergonomically ideal operating position (Stylopoulos & Rattner, 2003). Many studies highlighted that the operating surgeon experienced less physical strain with robotic assisted surgery (Stylopoulos & Rattner, 2003; Ballantyne et al., 2003; Hellan et al., 2007). In addition, robotic technology offers additional features such as motion scaling and remote telesurgical applications including tele-mentoring (Kim & Kang, 2010)

4.2 Limitations of the current robotic systems

The current robotic systems have some limitations which should be addressed in the future. There is lack of both tactile sensation and tensile feedback to the operating surgeon. Therefore, tissue damage can occur easily during traction by the robotic arm and during movement of the robotic instrument (Baik, 2008). Therefore, the surgeon must rely on visual cues to estimate the amount of tension exerted on the tissues (Hellan et al., 2007). Also, suture material can be cut during suturing because there is no tensile feedback to the robotic instrument (Baik, 2008). Therefore, great care must be taken to avoid traumatic injuries when handling bowel.

The system requires precise positioning of the robot for optimal operative outcome and to avoid robotic arm collision and the position of the patient cannot be changed without undocking the robotic arms (Hellan et al., 2007). The docking and separation procedure of a robotic cart from the patient is a time consuming procedure. Also, when using the robot to perform a surgical procedure in different compartments in the abdominal cavity, such as anterior resection, repeated docking and undocking of the robot is often needed and this is reflected on increased operating time. When immediate open conversion is necessary to deal with serious intra-operative bleeding delayed separation of the robotic cart can create a difficult situation (Baik, 2008).

High capital and running costs of the currently available robotic system made the taking up of this technology rather limited in many countries. The average price of one robotic system is more than U$2,000,000 and combining this with U$2,000 for the disposable instruments is a major issue when cost-effectiveness of robotic surgery is debated (Baik, 2008).

4.3 Approaches to robotic rectal surgery

There are several techniques for robotic rectal cancer surgery described in the surgical literature.

4.3.1 Multiple stages totally robotic technique

This is described as either a two-stage technique or a three-stage technique (D'Annibale et al., 2004). The number of stages mirrors the number of movements of the robotic cart. The need for frequent docking & undocking of the robotic system is reflected on increased operating time.

4.3.2 Hybrid technique

To eliminate the need for repositioning of the robot most surgeons choose conventional laparoscopic mobilization of the left colon and splenic flexure as well as division of the inferior mesenteric vessels and then use the robot for the TME part of the operation only. This hybrid approach saves the time for repetitive robotic setups. The actual TME is reported to take an average of 60 minutes (Hellan et al., 2007; Baik et al., 2008).

4.3.3 Single stage totally robotic

This approach has been recently reported by Kawak & Kim (2011). It eliminates the need for frequent docking & undocking of the robot but at the same time preserves the advantages of the use of the robotic approach for the whole procedure.

4.4 Advantages of totally robotic rectal surgery

Advocates of the totally robotic approach, whether multiple stage or single stage, believe that robotic dissection around the IMA pedicle is a fundamental step of the procedure to identify and preserve the periaortic nerves. They correctly consider that not only the pelvic nerves but also the periaortic nerves are important in sexual/bladder functions. They also feel that the use of robotics could also improve access and enable easier mobilization of the splenic flexure (Kawak & Kim, 2011).

4.5 Learning curve in robotic rectal surgery

The three-dimensional view and the ability of the robot to transfer the surgeon's hand movements to the tips of the surgical instruments makes the learning curve for robotic surgery much less steep than that for laparoscopic colorectal surgery. Therefore, an inexperienced laparoscopic surgeon is able to operate with the robot safely (Hellan et al, 2007). This is particularly evident for distal rectal cancers as the robot offers superior visualization and mobility during the pelvic dissection (Abodeely et al., 2010). Robotic surgery actually requires the same skill set used during open surgery and thus the learning curve at the console is relatively short (Giulianotti et al., 2003).

The learning curve of robotic assisted technology entails the surgeon's mastery of several unique skills to overcome the loss of tensile and tactile feedback by recognizing visual cues, conceptualize the spatial relationships of robotic instruments outside the active field of view and mentally visualizing the spatial relationships of the robotic arms and cart while operating at the console (Bokhari et al., 2011).

Bokhari et al. (2011) believe that to facilitate the acquisition of robotic unique skills in a safe and stepwise manner, the surgeon should acquire expert laparoscopic skills before using the robotic approach. They divided the learning curve into three phases. Phase 1 to include 15 cases and it represents the initial part of the learning curve. Phase 2 includes an additional 10 cases to allow the consolidation of the additional experience once the initial learning curve has been completed. Phase 3 is the post-learning period when the surgeon can start offering robotic surgery for a more complex and challenging cases. The authors concluded that their data suggest that after a learning curve phase that involves of 15 to 25 cases, the surgeon may achieve a higher level of competence and consider using robotic surgery for patients presenting with more difficult cases safely.

4.6 Outcomes of robotic assisted rectal surgery

4.6.1 Evidence from case series reports & case-matched studies

Pigazzi et al. (2006) reported the first series of robotic-assisted low anterior resection with total mesorectal excision on six consecutive patients with rectal cancer. These cases were compared with six consecutive low anterior resections performed with conventional laparoscopic technique by the same surgeon. There were no conversions in either group. Operative and pathological data, complications, and hospital stay were similar in both groups. However, robotic operations appeared to cause less strain for the operating surgeon. The authors concluded that robotic-assisted laparoscopic low anterior resection for rectal cancer is feasible in experienced hands and the technique may facilitate minimally invasive radical rectal surgery. The same group published 2 further case-matched reports with bigger series (Hellan et al., 2007; Baek et al., 2011) confirming their conclusion from the initial study. They particularly highlighted the low conversion rate with robotic assisted rectal surgery.

Patriti et al. (2009) reported on the short and medium term outcome of robotic assisted and traditional laparoscopic rectal resection in a case matched study. They found that robot-assisted laparoscopic rectal resection results in shorter operative time when a total mesorectal excision is performed and significantly lowers conversion rate. Postoperative morbidity was comparable between both groups. Overall survival and disease-free survival were comparable between groups, even though a trend towards better disease-free survival in the robotic assisted group was observed.

Baik et al. (2009) compared the short-term results between robotic-assisted low anterior resection and standard laparoscopic low anterior resection in rectal cancer. Conversion rate and serious complication rate were significantly lower in the robotic surgery group. The specimen quality was acceptable in both groups with a significantly better quality of the mesorectum grading in the robotic group.

Biffi et al. (2011) investigated the estimated blood loss after full robotic low anterior resection in a case-matched model with conventional open approach. Estimated intra-operative blood loss was significantly higher in the open group. They also found that the robotic surgery group had significantly decreased length of hospital stay, increased number of harvested lymph nodes and extent of distal margin.

Pigazzi et al. (2010) reported a multicentre study on the role of robot-assisted tumour-specific rectal surgery (RTSRS) to verify, on a multicentre basis, the peri-operative and oncologic outcome of RTSRS. The study included 140 consecutive patients undergoing RTSR in three centres. Conversion rate was 4. 9%. The number of harvested nodes and margin status compared favourably with those of open series. The 3-year overall survival rate was 97% with no isolated local recurrences were found at mean follow-up of 17. 4 months. The authors concluded that RTSRS is a safe and feasible procedure and highlighted the need for randomized clinical trials and longer follow-up are needed to evaluate a possible influence of RTSRS on patient survival.

Park et al. (2011) compared the short-term outcomes in 263 patients (open group = 88 patients, laparoscopic group n = 123 & robot-assisted group n = 52). Patients from the laparoscopic & robotic assisted groups recovered significantly faster than did those from the open surgery group. The specimen quality, with a distal resection margin, harvested lymph nodes, and circumferential margin, did not differ among the three groups. The authors concluded that laparoscopic & robotic assisted surgery reproduce equivalent short-term results of standard open surgery while providing the advantages of minimal access. For experienced laparoscopic colorectal surgeon, the use of the da Vinci robot resulted in no significant short-term clinical benefit over the conventional laparoscopic approach.

4.6.2 Evidence from randomised controlled trials (RCT)

There is lack of evidence from RCT to support robotic assisted surgery for rectal cancer. The **RO**botic versus **LA**paroscopic **R**esection for **R**ectal cancer **(ROLARR)** is designed to address this issue. This is an international, multicentre, prospective, randomised, controlled, unblinded, parallel-group trial of robotic-assisted versus laparoscopic surgery for the curative treatment of rectal cancer.

The study will perform a rigorous evaluation of robotic-assisted rectal cancer surgery against conventional laparoscopic rectal cancer resection by means of a randomised, controlled trial. Key short-term outcomes will include assessment of technical ease of the operation and improved oncological outcome. Also, quality of life assessment and analysis of cost-effectiveness will be performed. Short-term outcomes will be analysed to provide a timely assessment of the new technology. Longer-term outcomes will focus on oncological aspects of the disease with analysis of disease-free and overall survival and local recurrence rates at 3-year follow-up (http://www. leeds. ac. uk/hsphr/research/AUHE/rolarr. html).

5. Extended resection techniques in laparoscopic rectal cancer surgery

In an attempt to decrease the risk of local recurrence following radical surgery for rectal cancer, techniques have been described which offer extended resection. These were originally described in open surgery, but more recently these extended resections have been also offered laparoscopically (Georgiou et al., 2009; Stelzner et al., 2011).

5.1 Laparoscopic extended lateral pelvic node dissection

Lateral pelvic lymph node involvement in rectal cancer has been well recognised for many years (Sauer et al., 1951). In Japan, lateral pelvic node dissection is performed to minimise local recurrence and improve survival as they believe that total mesorectal excision does not clear the metastases in the lateral pelvic lymph nodes which has an overall incidence between 8. 6 to 27% (Fujita et al., 2003; Kim et al., 2008). However, evidence from meta-analysis confirms that extended lateral pelvic node dissection is associated with increased blood loss and urinary and sexual dysfunction without significant overall cancer-specific advantage (Georgiou et al., 2009). Therefore, preoperative radiotherapy or chemoradiotherapy followed by rectal resection with total mesorectal excision is the standard treatment in Western countries.

There is limited evidence in the literature on the outcomes of laparoscopic extended lateral pelvic node dissection with total meseorectal excision in patients with locally advanced rectal cancer. Advocates of the technique believe that laparoscopic approach has the potential to decrease the well known drawbacks of the open lateral pelvic wall dissection as the magnified views offer clear vision of the smallest structures in the narrow pelvis which make it easier to identify lymphatic tissue and protect the autonomic nerve plexus (Park et al., 2011). Some studies also suggest decreased blood loss and operative time with the laparoscopic approach (Fujita et al., 2003). Increasingly, robotic assisted approach has been used to perform extended lateral pelvic wall lymphadenectomy with remarks that dissection of the lymph nodes around major pelvic vessels is much easier (Park et al., 2011).

However, the currently available evidence is rather limited to make valid conclusions on the safety and outcomes of laparoscopic or robotic-assisted extended lateral pelvic node dissection in locally advanced rectal cancer.

5.2 Laparoscopic extended abdominoperineal resection for low rectal cancer

Standard abdominoperineal resection (APR) is well known to be associated with inferior oncological outcomes when compared to anterior resection for low rectal cancer (Stelzner et al., 2011). This is attributed to the relatively high incidence of intra-operative tumour or bowel perforation and positive circumferential resection margin due to the relative lack of the mesorectal fat around the lower rectum (Nagtegaal et al, 2005). This led to progressive development of an extended version of APR, now known as extended abdominoperineal resection (EAP), extralevator abdominoperineal excision (ELAP) or cylindrical abdominoperineal resection (Holm et al, 2007; Marecik et al, 2011). This technique aims at a wider circumferential resection margin at the level of the tumour bearing segment. Systematic reviews suggests that extended techniques of APR result in superior oncologic outcome in terms of lower incidence of tumour perforation and positive circumferential resection margin when compared to standard techniques (Stelzner et al., 2011).

However, extended abdominoperineal resection has been reported to be associated with higher incidence of perineal wound complications and hernia in comparison with the conventional APR. Also, lateral relatively blind excision of the levator muscles can put the neurovascular structures along the lateral pelvic wall at risk for injury which could increase the morbidity of the procedure. There are limited reports in the literature on laparoscopic and robotic assisted extended abdominoperineal resection (Marecik et al, 2011). However, the data so far are limited and more research is needed to assess the specific value of laparoscopic and robotic-assisted approach in relation to extended abdominoperineal resection.

6. Other approaches for laparoscopic rectal cancer surgery

There are few reports in the literature describing alternative approaches to rectal cancer surgey including single port access mesorectal excision (Gaujoux et al., 2011; Bulut et al., 2011; Lauritsen & Bulut, 2011), transanal or transvaginal retrieval of the specimen (Choi et al., 2009). However, the number of studies & cases are limited to make any valid conclusions. There is slow, but steadily increasing, interest in the application of completely natural orifice transluminal surgery (NOTES) in colorectal surgery (Sylla, 2010).

7. Conclusion

The debate over the optimal approach to the laparoscopic resection of rectal cancer is far from over. The short-term outcomes of conventional laparoscopic resections by experienced laparoscopic surgeons are better than those of open surgery and seem to be improving over time. The role of robotic assisted rectal surgery still needs to be better defined. There is limited evidence whether laparoscopic approach confers any long-term benefits for the patients. Also, further research is needed to establish if the different laparoscopic approaches can vary in their effect on the long term prognosis.

8. References

Abodeely, A.; Lagares-Garcia, J. A.; Duron, V.; Vrees M. (2010). Safety and learning curve in robotic colorectal surgery. J Robotic Surg; 4:161–165

Anderson, C.; Uman, G.; Pigazzi, A. (2008). Oncologic outcomes of laparoscopic surgery for rectal cancer: a systematic review and meta-analysis of the literature. Eur J Surg Oncol; 34(10)1135–42

Aziz, O.; Constantinides, V.; Tekkis, P.; et al. (2006). Laparoscopic versus open-surgery for rectal cancer: a meta-analysis. Ann Surg Onc;13:413–424

Baek, J. H.; Pastor, C.; Pigazzi, A. (2011). Robotic and laparoscopic total mesorectal excision for rectal cancer: a case-matched study. Surg Endosc; 25:521–525

Baik, S. H. (2008). Robotic colorectal surgery. Yonsei Med J.; 31; 49(6):891-6

Baik, S. H.; Lee, W. J.; Rha, K. H.; Kim, N. K.; Sohn, S. K.; Chi, H. S.; Cho, C. H.; Lee, S. K.; Cheon, J. H.; Ahn, J. B.; Kim, W. H. (2008). Robotic total mesorectal excision for rectal cancer using four robotic arms. Surg Endosc 22:792–797

Baik, S. H.; Kwon, H. Y.; Kim, J. S.; Hur, H; Sohn, S. K.; Cho, C. H.; Kim, H . (2009). Robotic versus laparoscopic low anterior resection of rectal cancer: short-term outcome of a prospective comparative study. Ann Surg Oncol.; 16(6):1480-7

Ballantyne, G. H.; Merola, P.; Weber, A.; Wasielewski, A. (2001). Robotic solutions to the pitfalls of laparoscopic colectomy. Osp Ital Chir;7:405-12

Ballantyne, G. H. (2002). Robotic surgery, telerobotic surgery, telepresence, and telementoring: review of early clinical results. Surg Endosc 16:1389–1402

Ballantyne, G. H.; Moll, F. (2003). The da Vinci telerobotic surgical system: the virtual operative field and telepresence surgery. Surg Clin North Am.; 83:1293–1304

Biffi, R.; Luca, F.; Pozzi, S.; Cenciarelli, S.; Valvo, M.; Sonzogni, A.; Radice, D.; Ghezzi, T. L. (2011). Operative blood loss and use of blood products after full robotic and conventional low anterior resection with total mesorectal excision for treatment of rectal cancer. J Robot Surg.; 5(2):101-107

Bokhari, M. B.; Patel, C. B.; Ramos-Valadez, D. I.; Ragupathi, M.; Haas, E. M.; (2011). Learning curve for robotic-assisted laparoscopic colorectal surgery. Surg Endosc.; 25(3):855-60

Brannigan, A. E.; De Buck, S.; Suetens, P.; Penninckx, F.; D'Hoore, A. (2006). Intracorporeal rectal stapling following laparoscopic total mesorectal excision: overcoming a challenge. Surg Endosc; 20: 952-955

Bretagnol, F.; Lelong, B.; Laurent, C.; et al. (2005). The oncological safety of laparoscopic total mesorectal excision with sphincter preservation for rectal carcinoma. Surg Endosc; 19 (7): 892–896

Breukink, S.; Pierie, J.; Wiggers, T. (2006). Laparoscopic versus open total mesorectal excision for rectal cancer. Cochrane Library, Cochrane Database of Systematic Reviews; 4:1–79

Bulut, O.; Nielsen, C. B.; Jespersen, N. (2011). Single-port access laparoscopic surgery for rectal cancer: initial experience with 10 cases. Dis Colon Rectum.; 54(7):803-9

Cecil, T. D.; Taffinder, N.; Gudgeon, A. M. (2006). A personal view on laparoscopic rectal cancer surgery. Colorectal Dis; 8: 30–2

Champagne, B. J.; Delaney, C. P. (2007). Laparoscopic approaches to rectal cancer. Clin Colon Rectal Surg; 20(3):237-48

Champagne, B. J.; Makhija, R. (2011). Minimally invasive surgery for rectal cancer: are we there yet? World J Gastroenterol; 17(7):862-6

Choi, D. H.; Hwang, J. K.; Ko, Y. T.; Jang, H. J.; Shin, H. K.; Lee, Y. C.; Lim, C. H.; Jeong, S. K.; Yang, H. K. (2010). Risk factors for anastomotic leakage after laparoscopic rectal resection. J Korean Soc Coloproctol.; 26(4):265-73

Choi, G. S.; Park, I. J.; Kang, B. M.; Lim, K. H.; Jun, S. H. (2009). A novel approach of robotic-assisted anterior resection with transanal or transvaginal retrieval of the specimen for colorectal cancer. Surg Endosc (2009) 23:2831–2835

D'Annibale, A.; Morpurgo, E.; Fiscon, V. et al. (2004) Robotic and laparoscopic surgery for treatment of colorectal diseases. Dis Colon Rectum 47:2162–2168

Delaney, C. P.; Lynch, A. G.; Senagore, A. J.; Fazio, V. W. (2003). Comparison of robotically performed and traditional laparoscopic colorectal surgery. Dis Colon Rectum; 46:1633-9

Enker, W. E.; Thaler, H. T.; Cranor, M. L.; Polyak, T. (1995). Total mesorectal excision in the operative treatment of carcinoma of the rectum. J Am Coll Surg; 181(4):335–346

Gaujoux, S.; Bretagnol, F.; Au, J.; Ferron, M.; Panis, Y. (2011). Single port access proctectomy with total mesorectal excision and intersphincteric resection with a primary transanal approach. Colorectal Dis.; 13(9):e305-7

Georgiou, P.; Tan, E.; Gouvas, N.; Antoniou, A.; Brown, G.; Nicholls, R. J.; Tekkis, P. (2009). Extended lymphadenectomy versus conventional surgery for rectal cancer: a meta-analysis. Lancet Oncol. 2009; 10:1053-62

Giulianotti, P. C.; Coratti, A.; Angelini, M.; et al. (2003). Robotics in general surgery: personal experience in a large community hospital. Arch Surg; 138:777–84

Good, D. W.; O'Riordan, J. M.; Moran, D.; Keane, F. B.; Eguare, E.; O'Riordain, D. S.; Neary, P. C. 2011. Laparoscopic surgery for rectal cancer: a single-centre experience of 120 cases. Int J Colorectal Dis. 2011 Jun 24. [Epub ahead of print]

Guillou, P. J.; Quirke, P.; Thorpe, H.; Walker, J.; Jayne, D. G.; Smith, A. M. et al. (2005). MRC CLASICC Trial Group. Short-term endpoints of conventional versus laparoscopicassisted surgery in patients with colorectal cancer (MRC CLASICC trial): multicentre, randomised controlled trial. Lancet; 365: 1718–26

Fujita, S.; Yamamoto, S.; Akasu, T.; Moriya, Y. (2003). Lateral pelvic lymph node dissection for advanced lower rectal cancer. Br J Surg; 90:1580–1585. Heald, R. J.; Ryall, R. D. (1986). Recurrence and survival after total mesorectal excision for rectal cancer. Lancet; 28; 1(8496):1479-82

Heald, R. J.; Moran, B. J.; Ryall, R. D.; Sexton, R.; MacFarlane, J. K. (1998). Rectal cancer: the Basingstoke experience of total mesorectal excision, 1978-1997. Arch Surg; 133(8):894–899

Hellan, M.; Anderson, C.; Ellenhorn, J. D.; Paz, B.; Pigazzi, A. (2007). Short-term outcomes after robotic-assisted total mesorectal excision for rectal cancer. Ann Surg Oncol.; 14(11):3168-73

Holm, T.; Ljung, A.; Häggmark, T.; Jurell, G.; Lagergren, J. (2007). Extended abdominoperineal resection with gluteus maximus flap reconstruction of the pelvic floor for rectal cancer. Br J Surg; 94:232–238

Ito, M.; Sugito, M.; Kobayashi, A.; Nishizawa, Y.; Tsunoda, Y.; Saito, N. (2008),. Relationship between multiple numbers of stapler firings during rectal division and anastomotic leakage after laparoscopic rectal resection. Int J Colorectal Dis; 23:703-7

Jacobs, M.; Verdeja, J. C.; Goldstein, H. S. (1991). Minimally invasive colon resection (laparoscopic colectomy). Surg Laparosc Endosc 1: 144–50

Kang, S. B.; Park, J. W.; Jeong, S. Y.; Nam, B. H.; Choi, H. S. et al (2010). Open versus laparoscopic surgery for mid or low rectal cancer after neoadjuvant chemoradiotherapy (COREAN trial): short-term outcomes of an open-label randomised controlled trial. Lancet Oncol.; 11(7):637-45

Kim, T. H.; Jeong, S. Y.; Choi, D. H.; Kim, D. Y.; Jung, K. H.; Moon, S. H.; Chang, H. J.; Lim, S. B.; Choi, H. S.; Park, J. G. (2008). Lateral lymph node metastasis is a major cause of locoregional recurrence in rectal cancer treated with preoperative chemoradiotherapy and curative resection. Ann Surg Oncol; 15:729–737

Kim, J. S.; Cho, S. Y.; Min, B. S.; Kim, N. K. (2009). Risk factors for anastomotic leakage after laparoscopic intracorporeal colorectal anastomosis with a double stapling technique. J Am Coll Surg; 209:694-701

Kim, N. K. & Kang, J. (2010). Optimal Total Mesorectal Excision for Rectal Cancer: the Role of Robotic Surgery from an Expert's View. J Korean Soc Coloproctol.; 26(6):377-87

Kwak, J. M., Kim, S. G. (2011). The technique of single-stage totally robotic low anterior resection. J Robotic Surg; 5:25–28

Lacy, A. M.; Garcia-Valdecasas, J. C.; Delgado, S.; Castells, A.; Taurá, P.; Piqué, J. M. et al. (2002). Laparoscopy-assisted colectomy versus open colectomy for treatment of nonmetastatic colon cancer: a randomized trial. Lancet; 359: 2224–9

Lanfranco, A. R.; Castellanos, A. E.; Desai, J. P.; Meyers, W. C. (2004). Robotic surgery: a current perspective. Ann Surg.; 239:14–21

Laurent, C.; Leblanc, F.; Gineste, C.; Saric, J.; Rullier, E. (2007). Laparoscopic approach in surgical treatment of rectal cancer. Br J Surg; 94(12):1555–61

Lauritsen, M. L.; Bulut, O. (2011). Single-port access laparoscopic abdominoperineal resection through the colostomy site: a case report. Tech Coloproctol. [Epub ahead of print]

Lee, S. W.; Sonoda, T.; Milsom, J. W. (2007). Expediting of laparoscopic rectal dissection using a hand-access device. Dis Colon Rectum ; 50(6):927–929

Lee, S. W. (2009). Laparoscopic Procedures for Colon and Rectal Cancer Surgery. Clin Colon Rectal Surg; 22:218–224

Leung, K. L.; Kwok, S. P. Y.; Lam, S. C. W.; et al. (2004). Laparoscopic resection of rectosigmoid carcinoma: prospective randomised trial. Lancet; 363: 1187–92

Li, S.; Chi, P.; Lin, H.; Lu, X.; Huang, Y. (2011). Long-term outcomes of laparoscopic surgery versus open resection for middle and lower rectal cancer: an NTCLES study. Surg Endosc. 2011 Apr 13. [Epub ahead of print]

Lujan, J.; Valero, G.; Hernandez, Q.; Sanchez, A.; Frutos, M. D.; Parrilla P. (2009). Randomized clinical trial comparing laparoscopic and open surgery in patients with rectal cancer. Br J Surg; 96: 982-989

Maeso S, Reza M, Mayol JA, Blasco JA, Guerra M, Andradas E, et al. (2010) Efficacy of the Da Vinci surgical system in abdominal surgery compared with that of laparoscopy: a systematic review and meta-analysis. Ann Surg.;252:254-62

Marecik, S. J.; Zawadzki, M.; Desouza, A. L.; Park, J. J.; Abcarian, H.; Prasad, L. M. (2011). Robotic cylindrical abdominoperineal resection with transabdominal levator transection. Dis Colon Rectum; 54:1320-5

Morino, M.; Parini, U.; Giraudo, G.; Salval, M.; Brachet Contul, R.; Garrone C. (2003). Laparoscopic total mesorectal excision: a consecutive series of 100 patients. Ann Surg; 237(3): 335–342

Nagtegaal, I. D.; van de Velde, C. J.; Marijnen, G. C.; van Krieken, J. H. J. M., Quirke, P. (2005). Low rectal cancer: a call for a change of approach in abdominoperineal resection. J Clin Oncol 23:9257–9264

Ng, K. H.; Ng, D. C.; Cheung, H. Y.; Wong, J. C.; Yau, K. K.; Chung, C. C.; Li, M. K. (2009). Laparoscopic resection for rectal cancers: lessons learned from 579 cases. Ann Surg; 249: 82-86

Ng, S. S.; Leung, K. L.; Lee, J. F.; Yiu, R. Y.; Li J. C.; Hon, S. S. (2009). Long-term morbidity and oncologic outcomes of laparoscopic-assisted anterior resection for upper rectal cancer: ten-year results of a prospective, randomized trial. Dis Colon Rectum; 52: 558-566

Park, J. S.; Choi, G. S.; Lim, K. H.; Jang, Y. S.; Jun, S. H. (2011). S052: a comparison of robot-assisted, laparoscopic, and open surgery in the treatment of rectal cancer. Surg Endosc.; 25(1):240-8

Patriti, A.; Ceccarelli, G.; Bartoli, A.; Spaziani, A.; Biancafarina, A.; Casciola, L. (2009). Short- and medium-term outcome of robot-assisted and traditional laparoscopic rectal resection. JSLS.; 13(2):176-83

Pigazzi, A.; Ellenhorn, J. D.; Ballantyne, G. H.; Paz, I. B. (2006). Roboticassisted laparoscopic low anterior resection with total mesorectal excision for rectal cancer. Surg Endosc; 20:1521-5

Pigazzi, A.; Luca, F.; Patriti, A.; Valvo, M.; Ceccarelli, G.; Casciola, L.; Biffi, R.; Garcia-Aguilar, J.; Baek, J. H. (2010). Multicentric study on robotic tumor-specific mesorectal excision for the treatment of rectal cancer. Ann Surg Oncol.; 17(6):1614-20

Quah, H. M.; Jayne, D. G.; Eu, K. W.; Seow-Choen, F. (2002). Bladder and sexual dysfunction following laparoscopically assisted and conventional open mesorectal resection for cancer. Br J Surg; 89:1551–1556

Quirke, P.; Dixon, M. F. (1988). The prediction of local recurrence in rectal adenocarcinoma by histopathological examination. Int J Colorectal Dis.; 3(2):127-31

Sauer, I.; Bacon, H. E. (1951). Influence of lateral spread of cancer of the rectum on radicability of operation and prognosis. Am J Surg; 81:111–120

Scheidbach, H.; Schneider, C.; Konradt, J. et al. (2002). Laparoscopic abdominoperineal resection and anterior resection with curative intent for carcinoma of the rectum. Surg Endosc; 16:7–13

Shalli, K.; MacDonald, E.; Aly, E. H. (2009). Towards lower complication rate in laparoscopic rectal surgery. Colorectal Disease, 11 (Suppl. 2), 55. Abstract

Simons, A. J.; Anthone, G. J.; Ortega, A. E.; et al. (1995). Laparoscopic-assisted colectomy learning curve. Dis Colon Rectum; 38: 600–03

Stelzner, S.; Koehler, C.; Stelzer, J.; Sims, A.; Witzigmann, H. (2011). Extended abdominoperineal excision vs. standard abdominoperineal excision in rectal cancer-a systematic overview. Int J Colorectal Dis.; 26(10):1227-40

Stylopoulos, N.; Rattner, D. (2003). Robotics and ergonomics. Surg Clin North Am.; 83:1321–37

Sylla; P. (2010). Current experience and future directions of completely NOTES colorectal resection. World J Gastrointest Surg.; 2(6): 193-198

Tekkis; P. P.; Senagore; A. J.; Delaney, C. P., Fazio, V. W. (2005). Evaluation of the learning curve in laparoscopic colorectal surgery: comparison of right-sided and left-sided resections. Ann Surg; 242(1):83–91

Veldkamp, R.; Kuhry, E.; Hop, W. C.; Jeekel, J.; Kazemier, G.; Bonjer, H. J. et al. (2005). Colon cancer Laparoscopic or Open Resection Study Group (COLOR). Laparoscopic surgery versus open surgery for colon cancer: short-term outcomes of a randomised trial. Lancet Oncol; 6: 477–84

Vithiananthan, S.; Cooper, Z.; Betten, K.; et al. (2001). Hybrid laparoscopic flexure takedown and open procedure for rectal resection is associated with significantly shorter length of stay than equivalent open resection. Dis Colon Rectum; 44(7):927–935

Zhu, Q. L.; Feng, B.; Lu, A. G.; Wang, M. L.; Hu, W. G.; Li, J. W.; Mao, Z. H.; Zheng, M. H. (2010). Laparoscopic low anterior resection for rectal carcinoma: complications and management in 132 consecutive patients. World J Gastroenterol.; 16(36):4605-10

Part 3

Emergency Colorectal Surgery

4

Emergency Surgery for Colorectal Cancer Complications: Obstruction, Perforation, Bleeding

Gelu Osian
University of Medicine and Pharmacy "Iuliu Hatieganu" Cluj-Napoca
Romania

1. Introduction

Colorectal cancer represents the third most common cause of malignancy in men and the fourth most common cause of malignancy in women. Prevalence is estimated at 25 to 100,000 inhabitants (1).

Left colon cancer is more frequent than right colon cancer with half of colorectal cancers being situated at the level of the sigmoid colon.

There is a higher incidence of this form of malignancy in developed countries with higher living and is thought to be mainly due to environmental factors. An improvement in survival of the patients has been obtained thanks to national screening programs which enables diagnosis in the early stages which allows for treatment.

Despite current screening guidelines a large number of cases present to the surgical clinic as complications of colorectal cancer in the advanced, such as are tumoral obstruction, colon perforation, and lower GI hemorrhage.

The age of patients presenting with these complications is generally advanced, a factor which contributes to a high post-operative mortality of patients. Malignant processes evolve over a longer period in order for these complications to be produced, which is why patients are usually found to be in advanced stages of oncologic evolution with peritoneal carcinomatosis or distance metastasis. Despite this fact, radical treatment for the complicated colorectal cancer is recommended whenever possible.

2. Obstruction from colorectal cancer

The great majority of colorectal cancers have an asymptomatic or paucisymptomatic evolution over an extended period of time until they succeed in being clinically determined by a major complication. This is often a lower intestinal occlusion. Several cases have been cited whereby patients have beencompletely asymptomatic but have a sudden clinical onset. This was reported as a result of air flights, but without establishing a correlation between the flight and onset of disease (2).

Of the total colorectal cancers (CRC) 8-10% present as bowel occlusions, their variability being registered depending on the specificity of the surgical service. They do not tend to have a favorable prognosis due to the increased age of patients, the advanced stage and the emergency nature of the surgical intervention (3).

Cancer represents the most frequent cause of large bowel obstruction, comprising 60% of the occlusions in elderly patients. Two thirds of colorectal cancers are situated at the left colon level and one third at right colon level (4).

Intestinal occlusion due to CRC has always raised problems regarding surgical treatment. Due to the fact that most of these patients are operated as an emergency, their metabolic state is insufficiently assessed and mechanically, the colon is not ready for surgical intervention. Surgical teams must make an ongoing choice between surgical treatments in one operative session and serialized surgical interventions. At present the most common choice is usually made for resection with primary anastomosis (5).

2.1 Presentation

Patients present to surgical clinic with abdominal colic pains, abdominal distension, altered mental status, and cessation of bowel transit of gas and feces. The patient is usually elderly, with altered general state, signs of neoplastic toxicity, and rich hyperseptic colon content.

As opposed to small bowel occlusions, colic-like pains are less frequent and less intense. Intestinal distension comprises solely the colic framework for a long period of time and only later does it extend to the small bowel. At this point, fecal vomiting occurs. The mechanism of vomiting is through a a reflex mechanism present in abdominal colic. On exam, distension of the abdomen on the colic frame shows dullness on percussion. In older occlusions, distension with dullness comprises the whole abdomen.

The abdomen is slightly sensitive spontaneously and to palpation. On auscultation, can be noted accentuated bowel sounds are detected. In older occlusive forms, the absence of sounds due to the presence of paralytic ileus.

At the per rectum examination, an empty rectal ampule is detected, without fecal matter. Quite often in lower rectal cancers, the tumor, which is completely stenotic, may be palpated by the exploratory finger.

Following fecal vomiting and abdominal fluid sequestration, the patient shows signs of dehydration and shock with cold, cyanotic, dried teguments and low blood pressure .

2.2 Diagnosis

Abdominal X-ray emphasizes few hydro-aeric levels situated in the colonic frame, and having a large diameter vertically. This investigation can therefore make a diagnosis of a large bowel obstruction. Abdominal ultrasound shows dilated intestinal loops with liquid content and bracing movements. It can also reveal free liquid in the peritoneal cavity, can highlight the mass formed at the colon level if it is of significant size and can also observe potential metastatic disseminations to other abdominal organs.

Abdominal CT diagnoses the obstruction and can detect the primary tumor with its potential secondary determinations with a greater precision than abdominal ultrasound.

When the general state of the patients enables, a colonoscopy can be performed, highlighting the colorectal cancer, taking a biopsy and also perform potential trans-tumoral drilling which can relieve the obstruction with the possibility of a delayed emergency surgical intervention.

A chest X Ray can also detect potential secondary pulmonary metastasis.

Due to the older age of patients and their multiple co-morbidities, an extensive pre-operative assessment is necessary, measuring creatinine, urea and electrolytes and arterial blood gases. Patients are usually dehydrated suffering from severe metabolic imbalances which must be treated at the preoperative stage.

The ECG is Compulsory part of the surgical preoperative protocol.

2.3 Differential diagnosis

A diagnosis of large bowel obstruction can be made with the aid of history taking, the objective examination, and also the additional investigations performed. However, a differential diagnosis is required mainly having to rule out small bowel obstructions with higher intestinal occlusions. These usually determine a more painful and prominent symptomatology, with more frequent and intense colicky pains, with frequent food vomiting and only later, in neglected obstructions, they become fecaloid. Abdominal X Ray highlights hydroaeric levels with central disposition, having a large diameter on the horizontal plane. Other causes must also be ruled out including intussusception, sigmoid volvulus, engagement of the colon in a hernia sac with strangulation, invasion of the colon in the framework of extension of a neoplastic process from proximity (stomach, genital, urinary, pancreas etc).

Once the tumoral cause of the obstruction is established, a differential diagnosis of causes of colonic tumors is necessary, namely stenosed vegetating benign tumors, phytobezoar etc. Often the decision for surgical treatment is made in an emergency and the final diagnosis is only made intra-operative.

2.4 Preoperative treatment

Preoperative assessment and treatment must be carefully and rapidly undertaken, in order to avoid delay of a surgical intervention in patients who may have altered mental status or unstable vital signs. Metabolic acidosis, hypo or hyperglycemia and electrolyte imbalances are corrected based on the previous investigations performed. Antibiotics are administered prophylactically at this stage and the choice is usually a second or third generation cephalosporin in conjuction with Metronizadole or Vancomycin. Also, prophylaxis of deep venous thrombosis prophylaxis is achieved with low molecular weight heparin. Symptomatic treatment may be given to relieve the distress and may includes, analgesics, antiemetics, gastric antisecretion drugs and anticholinergics (6).

Oral laxatives are contra indicated.

If there is a probability that the surgical intervention includes a colostomy, it is advisable to mark the pre-operated place of colostomy.

All other co-morbidities must be optimized whenever possible.

2.5 Treatment options

In the therapeutic strategy of obstructive colorectal cancer, application of palliative methods and other radical treatment methods are advised.. Whenever possible, treatment has to be radical.

Palliative treatment is recommended in patients with severely altered general health and advanced stage disease with hepatic non- resectable metastasis (7).

Palliative treatment can be carried out as follows: pneumatic dilation of the tumorally stenosed region with the help of a balloon or rechanneling with laser Nd-YAG which can be effective as a palliative method in 80-90% of patients.

Endoscopic setting of the auto expandable metallic prosthesis has been used more and more with greater success in the preparation of the radical or palliative surgery for a non-resectable obstructive cancer. If this procedure is performed by an experienced surgeon, the success rate is over 90% (8).

In the operable cases, the implanted stent allows the gastrointestinal transit to restart while resolving the obstruction at the same time. Subsequently, the patient's condition and biological parameters improve, also permitting the delivery of neoadjuvant therapy where needed (9).

The affected bowel reduces its dimensions, the edema disappears and blood perfusion to the bowel improves. All of these changes create the premise for a planned radical intervention to be performed. A study done by Tekkis (8) looked at two groups of patients with obstructive colon cancer and similar tumor stages. One group had an initial surgical treatment and the other group had the endoscopic prosthesis as a first step followed by a surgical intervention. In the group who received the stent prosthesis, there were 87% of cases who ended up having resection and anastomosis, compared to 41% of cases in the non-stented group.

The specific complications associated with stoma care have to be considered, as they potentially increase co-morbidities, hospital admission, and also the costs of the intervention. The post-operative evolution was better in the group of patients who received the endoscopic stent, and they also had a shorted hospital admission (8). Performing elective surgical interventions also proved to decrease post-operatory mortality.

Inserting expandable metallic stents is the intervention of choice for tumors in the advanced stages, with metastasis and peritoneal carcinomatosis.

A study done by Jeffrey H. Lee et al (10) showed that this method is safe and feasible. When it was performed by an experienced team, it had a success rate of 94%. Re-obstruction caused by the tumoral proliferation was noted in 7.3% cases. Death occurred due to specific complications related to the neoplastic process rather than surgical interventions.

Some of the disadvantages of the stenting process are related to the iatrogenic complications as a result of inserting the prosthesis in emergency conditions. Watt et al (11) noted that the rate of complications was of 27%. These include stent migration (11%), perforation (4.5%) and tumoral growth with stent obstruction (12%).

Radical treatment can be performed during a surgical intervention or during serialized interventions. In the course of history, the following were performed: at the end of the 19th century Paul-Mikulicz performed the intervention in one single operative session through externalizing the colon together with the tumor, which was resected postoperatively and an external anastomosis with a special clamp was performed. This operation was performed in one single intervention and has the advantage of lowering operative mortality by 70% compared to previous procedures, but also has the disadvantage of a high local recurrence. At the beginning of the 20th century the procedure used was one completed in three separate interventions:

1. colostomy which resolved the occlusion,
2. resection of the tumor and ultimately
3. restoring the intestinal transit. The advantage of this method is that it was performed on a mechanically stable colon but had the great disadvantage of a high morbidity rate of 30% (30% the morbidity rate) and mortality of 7% for each operative intervention In 1921, Hartmann proposed a procedure divided into two phases resection of the tumor with terminal colostomy subsequently followed by restoring of the intestinal transit. The advantage consists of rapid removal of the tumor and resolving the occlusion. The anastomosis is not performed on unfavorable terms, but the disadvantage is that of summation of mortality and morbidity indexes for each operative session, given that reintegration in transit is made through a new laparotomy.

The objective of analyzing the historical data was to avoid serialized operative disadvantages and surgical intervention in one operative session with primary anastomosis as the preferred option (12), (13).

2.6 Surgical options in obstructive colorectal cancers

Surgical attitude is different depending on the localization of tumor.

In right colon cancers the indicated operation is right hemicolectomy with primary ileotransverse anastomosis. In elderly patients with increasing age, a significantly altered general state or peritoneal carcinomatosis, the accepted operation is ileotransverse anastomosis with short circuiting of the tumoral obstacle.

In transverse colon cancers, the unanimously accepted surgical intervention is the single resection with a primary anastomosis. In special cases with very significant colon distension, elderly patients with multiple organic deficiencies, a very altered general state or peritoneal carcinomatosis, two phases are indicated for the intervention: colostomy immediately upwards from the tumor then followed by segmentary resection with colo-colonic anastomosis.

Cancers localized to the left colon level have the greatest number of controversies regarding operations in a single session or in two sessions. It is ideal to have a left hemicolectomy with primary colo-rectal anastomosis. If there is an insufficient preparation of the colon, there is a leakage at the hydro-pneumatic test, or anastomosis tension, a protection colostomy is recommended for execution or a provisional ileostomy. If there is severe distension of the colon, technical difficulties in resecting the tumor or ASA (American Society of Anesthesiologists) score >3 (high operative risk), a two step surgical intervention is recommended. The primary step consists of a colostomy, which frees the patient from occlusion, or Hartmann type operation, and resection with anastomosis, or anstomosis as secondary step, respectively. Due to the fact that many patients with left colon cancer are admitted for surgical intervention with an obstruction which evolves over a longer period and therefore there is marked distension of the entire colonic frame, in such cases subtotal colectomy with primary anastomosis was proposed. The advantages of the procedure consisted of removing potential synchronous cancers which were left undiagnosed at the preoperative stage due to the urgent nature of the surgical intervention. Also there is a small risk of fistula for the ileo-colonic anastomosis, similar to that of elective surgery,. The procedure eliminates the necessity for post operative follow-up colonoscopy. Disadvantages consist of extending the surgical intervention with a subsequent increase in operative risk and in the presence of numerous stools postoperatively. There are still a multitude of controversies regarding the treatment of such lesions.

In rectal cancers surgical attitude is dictated by the patient's general state, localization and oncologic stage of the tumor. Either an anterior rectum resection of the tumor with primary anastomosis, a Hartmann operation or a simple colostomy can be performed.

2.7 Postoperative treatment

At the post operative stage, intensive rebalancing of the patient is continued, low molecular weight heparin is administered prophylactically to prevent thromboembolic complications and a further prophylactic dose of antibiotic is administered.

Drainage disturbances are monitored and suppressed as early as possible. Nutrition with liquid intake is restarted upon resolution of the ileus, followed by solid food once intestinal transit is restored.

Skin threads are suppressed 7 to 10 days post operatively.

The results of surgical treatment are less effective because they are performed in emergency situations and add multiple surgical risk factors. In 2005, Coco detected a 44% morbidity and a 4% mortality in emergency surgery of these tumors compared to 12% morbidity and 0% mortality in the elective surgery of the of tumors in the same locations (14).

Zhang MS and his collaborators (15) highlighted the fact that the prognosis of patients with occlusive neoplasms of the left colon and of the rectum depends on the TNM stage of the disease, the preoperative level of CEA, and the radical nature of the surgical intervention.

Localization of the occlusive tumor does not influence the prognosis (16).

2.8 Personal experience

In the Surgery Clinic No III from Cluj-Napoca, the treatment approach of occlusive colorectal cancers is surgical. In all situations where the disease is potentially treatable and the general and local state of the patient enables, resection is performed within oncologic safety limits as well as regional lymphadenectomy with reconstruction of continuity through primary anastomosis. If the bowel is highly distended and edematous, a Hartmann type intervention is performed or a resection with anastomosis and protective ileostomosis. In patients with severely altered general state, in those with a surgically surpassed disease, an upward colostomy or internal derivation is performed.

2.9 Conclusion

Occlusive colorectal cancers are severe forms of disease which represent a serious problem of therapeutic strategy, that is still intensely debated at present. Whenever possible, a radical surgical treatment is indicated with a single operative resection and primary anastomosis.

3. Perforated CRC

The incidence of perforated colorectal cancer is approximately 2.3-2.5% of the total number of surgically treated colorectal cancers (3). This is not a very common complication; however it is very serious due to the severe peritonitis that results. Perforations of the colon have been documented in the literature after administration of bevacizumab for malignant tumors of the colon (17).

3.1 Introduction

Colorectal cancer can present emergently as a colonic perforation as a result of leakage of the hyperseptic content into the peritoneal cavity and subsequently causing localized or generalized peritonitis. The perforation can be produced in a juxtatumoral position or or at some distance from the tumor, the so-called diastatic perforation. It usually appears in large neoplasms which evolve over a longer period of time, being therefore advanced from a regional perspective. Diastatic perforation appears in left colon cancers which undergo complete stenosis and result in upwards colon distension. The vascularization of the cecum where the perforation occurs, results in the outflow of the hyperseptic stasis content into the peritoneal cavity with consecutive peritonitis. Juxtatumoral perforation appears most frequently in right colon cancers and causes an abscess which subsequently perforates into the free peritoneum.

Tumoral perforation appears in the advanced stages of the disease. In the study conducted by Masaichi Ogawa and his collaborators (18) it is shown that in 53% of cases the disease is in stage IV, while in 37% it is in stage IIIb and in 10% stage IIIa.

3.2 Presentation

Patients are referred to the hospital showing signs of an acute surgical abdomen. Abdominal pain is intense and diffused with low blood pressure, cold cyanotic teguments, and altered general health state. The history taking reveals colon distress manifested as diarrhea alternating with constipation, weight loss and stools with blood, mucus and pus.

On exam, patients can show signs of septic shock, with general abdominal muscular contraction and peritoneal irritation. In the later stages they can present with a distended abdomen without intestinal peristalsis with an intensely altered general state and signs of shock.

In the case of intra peritoneal abscess which has not yet opened into the entire peritoneal cavity, signs of peritonitis are localized at the tumor level which may be palpated on exam. If the perforation has led to the formation of a retroperitoneal abscess, the patient usually presents with a septic state associated to subcutaneous emphysema and abdominal wall cellulites.

3.3 Diagnosis

The diagnosis is mainly clinical and demands urgent surgical treatment.

Abdominal X-rays display pneumoperitoneum in the case of free perforation in the peritoneal cavity. Marked cecum distension can be discerned with diastatic perforation imminence even before its onset.

X-rays and abdominal CT scan show a consecutive intraperitoneal abscess in the blocked tumor perforation. Laboratory investigations reveal an important leukocytosis with potential signs of secondary renal failure from the emergent peritonitis.

3.4 Differential diagnosis

The juxtatumoral perforation of the cecum with consecutive abscess must be distinguished from a gangrenous and blocked appendicitis. This situation is especially due to the fact that this form of appendicitis can be seen in the elderly patients. In addition to cancer of the cecum may present in this manner. The ultimate diagnosis can often be established only after the histopathological examination of the surgical resection piece.

Perforated cancer of the sigmoid colon must be differentiated from perforated sigmoid diverticulitis with abscess, which often presents with a similar clinical picture. In this case too, the final diagnosis is histopathological.

Retroperitoneal abscess following perforation of left or right colon cancer must be differentiated from a retroperitoneal abscesses of renal origin. This differentiation can be performed following imaging explorations which reveal renal modifications.

3.5 Preoperatory preparation

The preoperative preparation needs to be short but thorough insofar as generalized peritonitis is concerned, so as not to delay the surgical intervention and miss the appropriate moment for surgical intervention. Shock therefore needs to be treatedand patients require a wide spectrum antibiotic prophylaxis, and finally basic preoperatory protocols (ECG, biochemistry, arterial blood gases, chest X-ray, etc).

3.6 Treatment

Due to the neoplastic background on which the hyperseptic peritonitis occurs, any large-scale surgical intervention resulting in anastomosis must be avoided as it is shown to have poor outcomes.

It is crucial for the treatment to be marked as high emergency. Together with the extended resections, this can improve the prognosis (19).

Treatment of the peritonitis mainly consists of abundant washing of the peritoneal cavity, multiple drains, and broad spectrum antibiotics.

The approach of the perforated tumor is different depending on the local situation. If it can be removedeasily, that can be done without an anastomosis, and instead through an upward terminal colostomy with closure of the remaining distal end (Hartmann type intervention) (20). If the tumor cannot be easily resected, a simple upwards derivative colostomy is performed or an ileostomy associated with the aforementioned peritonitis treatment. After the general condition of the patient improves, surgical intervention is performed and completed to remove the perforated tumor, if possible.

In case of diastatic perforation of the cecum, surgical treatment is a subtotal colectomy with ileostomy followed by the reconstruction of intestinal transit through an ileocolic or ileorectal anastomosis when the patient's condition improves.

3.7 Postoperative treatment

In the postoperatory stage, the antibiotic treatment of peritonitis continues, as well as the hydroelectrolythic and acid-base rebalancing as and venous thrombosis. Drains and colostomies are monitored and drains should be discontinued when deemed appropriate.

An improved survival rate at 5 years is associated with administration of postoperative chemotherapy, compared with patients who did not receive this following release from hospital (21).

3.8 Prognosis

Prognosis of this complication is linked to the evolution and stage of tumor and to the severity of the peritonitis. In general, this complication carries an unfavorable prognosis, especially in case of diastatic perforation (22).

Mortality reaches 30 to 40% in cases of tumor perforation. In cases of diastatic perforation, mortality is between 50% and 68% (23), (24). If cases of death are excluded shortly after the intervention, the prognosis of perforated colorectal cancers is similar to that of unperforated cancers in the same stage (25).

4. Colorectal haemorrhagic cancers

4.1 Introduction

Hemorrhagic cancers are those cancers of the rectum and colon which manifest as colorectal bleeding. This is usually presents as melena for those cancers situated at the right colon level or as rectorrhagia with fresh blood for those situated in more distal positions, especially those situated at the recto-sigmoid level (1). Cancers that present as severe hemorrhage are rare; but they usually manifest through rectorrhagia and are extremely critical (26). Such cases require emergency surgery due to hemorrhage and the immediate goal of the treatment is obtaining hemostasis. Radical treatment of colorectal cancer is encouraged whenever possible.

4.2 History

The patient is referred to a physician in order to determine the presence of blood in the stool, either as dark stool (melena), or as fresh blood. Symptoms usually appear in a patient with previous stool disturbances, with alternating diarrhea-constipation, weight loss over a couple of months and altered general condition. The patient also may have a history of abdominal pains often colicky-like. For recto-sigmoid cancers the patient can present with rectal tenesmus and pathological products in the stool (eg. mucus). Usually patients are pale and frail, showing signs of acute or chronic anemia. At the rectal examination, fecal occult blood may be detected.

4.3 Diagnosis

In the presence of lower gastro-intestinal hemorrhage, colonoscopy is performed and highlights the presence of colorectal cancer with localization of the hemorrhagic source. Biopsies are collected for the histopathological diagnosis. Abdominal ultrasound and CT scan establishes the lesional abdominal record by emphasizing the local and regional extension of the lesion. Pulmonary radiologic exploration detects any eventual pulmonary disseminations of the colorectal cancer.

The TC99 scintigraphy has a reliability of 100% and a sensitivity of 91% in establishing the source of hemorrhage (27).

Biochemical and hematological explorations are compulsory for the preoperatory inventory. Microcytic hypochromic anemia is usually detected, requiring preoperatory correction with blood transfusion.

4.4 Differential diagnosis

A differential diagnosis has to be made between lower and upper gastro-intestinal tract hemorrhage. Upper digestive hemorrhage originates above the ligament of Treitz and it is usually manifested through hematemesis and melena. If the hemorrhage is significant it can manifest itself as a rectorrhagia, but is usually associated with hematemesis. Emergency colonoscopy branches out the diagnosis. Apart from colorectal cancer there are other diseases which can evolve with rectorrhagia, for example ulcero-hemorrhagic rectocolitis, benign tumors which can cause bleeding, intestinal mesenteric infarct, intestinal invagination, etc. However, the clinical picture is different to that of colorectal cancer, as there can be present signs of peritonitis and shock (intestinal-mesenteric infarct) or of bowel obstruction (invagination). At the distal gastro-intestinal tract, the cause of rectorrhagia can be represented by hemorrhoids or anal fissure, which can be detected through anoscopy and rectal examination.

4.5 Preoperative treatment

The preoperative assessment and treatment is usually performed as an emergency in order not to delay surgical intervention. Correction of anemia is necessary through transfusion of packed red blood cells, often rh- because of the emergent nature.

Electrolytes should be monitored and corrected as appropriate.

4.6 Treatment

The objective is to remove the source of hemorrhage, i.e. the source of colorectal cancer. If possible, an intervention with radical aim is performed when the patient's general condition allows it.

Therefore, in right colon hemorrhagic cancers a right hemicolectomy is performed, while in left colon cancers a left hemicolectomy. In recto-sigmoid cancers a resection or rectum amputation is planned depending on the distance from the tumor to the anal margin.

There are situations when the cancer is in the advanced stages, making it impossible to be removed. In these cases a derivative process can be performed with anupward colostomy type or the colo-colonic or entero-colonic derivation thus putting the colon to rest in the hope that in the absence of local trauma represented by the fecal discharge, the hemorrhage will stop.

4.7 Postoperatory treatment

Resuscitation procedures initiated at the pre operatory stage are continued with whole blood transfusions or packed red blood cells and prophylactic antibiotics aiming to correct the hemorrhagic shock.

The stoma and the surgical trauma are appropriately treated.

4.8 Results and prognosis

These depend on the stage of evolution of the colorectal cancer and advanced forms with marked regional invasion have a poor prognosis.

5. Conclusions

Fortunately, complicated colorectal cancers with significant hemorrhage are rare. They usually present with occult bleeding and chronic signs of anemia.. The advanced regional forms with severe hemorrhage from the necrosed tumor unfortunately have little therapeutic options and results are poor.

6. References

[1] Osian G. Cancerul colorectal-De la Genetica la Chirurgia Robotica. Editura Medicala Universitara Iuliu Hatieganu 2011. pp 116-120.

[2] Kingsley C Ekwueme, Malcolm A West, Paul S Rooney. Emergency first presentation of colorectal cancer following air travel: a case series J R Soc Med Sh Rep May 2011 2:36; doi:10.1258/shorts.2011.011002

[3] Beuran M., Grigorescu M. Actualitati in patologia colonului. Editura Medicala Universitara Iuliu Hatieganu 2007. pp.68-72.

[4] Kronborg O., Backer O., Sprechler M. Acute obstruction in cancer of the colon and rectum. Dis colon Rectum 1975; 18: 22-27.

[5] Smithers BM, Theile D.E., Cohen JR.,et al. Emergency surgery for obstructing colorectal cancers: a comparison between right-sided and left-sided lesions. J AM Coll Surg 2001; 193(6): 717.

[6] O'Connor B, Creedon B. Pharmacological treatment of bowel obstruction in cancer patients. Expert Opin Pharmacother. 2011 Oct;12(14):2205-14. Epub 2011 Jun 30.

[7] Dalal KM, Gollub MJ, Miner TJ, Wong WD, Gerdes H, Schattner MA, Jaques DP, Temple LK. Management of patients with malignant bowel obstruction and stage IV colorectal cancer. J Palliat Med. 2011 Jul;14(7):822-8. Epub 2011 May 19.

[8] P. P. Tekkis, J. D. Poloniecki, M. R. Thompson, J. D. Stamatakis. Operative mortality in colorectal cancer: prospective national study. British Medical Journal, vol. 327, no. 7425, pp. 1196–1199, 2003.

[9] D. Williams,1 R. Law,2 and A. M. Pullyblank. Colorectal Stenting in Malignant Large Bowel Obstruction: The Learning Curve. International Journal of Surgical Oncology.vol 2011 (2011), Article ID 917848, 4 pages doi:10.1155/2011/917848

[10] Jeffrey H. Lee, William A. Ross, Raquel Davila, George Chang, E. Lin, Alexander Dekovich and Marta Davila. Self-Expandable Metal Stents (SEMS) Can Serve as a Bridge to Surgery or as a Definitive Therapy in Patients with an Advanced Stage of Cancer: Clinical Experience of a Tertiary Cancer Center. Digestive Diseases and Sciences. vol. 55, no. 12, pp. 3530-3536, 2010.

[11] A. M. Watt, I. G. Faragher, T. T. Griffin, N. A. Rieger, and G. J. Maddern. Self-expanding metallic stents for relieving malignant colorectal obstruction: a systematic review. Annals of Surgery, vol. 246, no. 1, pp. 24–30, 2007.

[12] Ansaloni L, Andersson RE, Bazzoli F, Catena F, Cennamo V, Di Saverio S, Fuccio L, Jeekel H, Leppäniemi A, Moore E, Pinna AD, Pisano M, Repici A, Sugarbaker PH, Tuech JJ. Guidelenines in the management of obstructing cancer of the left colon: consensus conference of the world society of emergency surgery (WSES) and peritoneum and surgery (PnS) society. World J Emerg Surg. 2010 Dec 28;5:29.

[13] Sasaki K, Kazama S, Sunami E, Tsuno NH, Nozawa H, Nagawa H, Kitayama J.One-stage segmental colectomy and primary anastomosis after intraoperative colonic irrigation and total colonoscopy for patients with obstruction due to left-sided colorectal cancer. Dis Colon Rectum. 2012 Jan;55(1):72-8

[14] Claudio Coco, Alessandro Verbo, Alberto Manno, Claudio Mattana, Marcello Covino, Giorgio Pedretti, Luigi Petito, Gianluca Rizzo and Aurelio Picciocchi. Impact of Emergency Surgery in the Outcome of Rectal and Left Colon Carcinoma. World J Surg (2005) 29: 1458–1464.

[15] Zhang MS, Mao WZ, Zhou YB, Wang PG, Zhang BY. Surgical treatment and prognostic factors for obstructing left colorectal cancer. Zhonghua Wei Chang Wai Ke Za Zhi 2011 Aug; 14(8):620-622.

[16] Frago R, Biondo S, Millan M, Kreisler E, Golda T, Fraccalvieri D, Miguel B, Jaurrieta E . Differences between proximal and distal obstructing colonic cancer after curative surgery. Colorectal Dis 2011 Jun; 13(6):e116-22.

[17] Bevacizumab-induced bowel perforation.Sliesoraitis S, Tawfik B. J Am Osteopath Assoc. 2011 Jul;111(7):437-41.

[18] Masaichi Ogawa, Michiaki Watanabe, Ken Eto, Takahiro Omachi, Makoto Kosuge, … Ken Hanyu, Lohta Noaki, Tetsuji Fujita, Katsuhiko Yanaga. Clinicopathological features of perforated colorectal cancer._Anticancer Research (2009) Volume: 29, Issue: 5, Pages: 1681-1684.

[19] Carraro PG, Segala M, Orlotti C, Tiberio G. Outcome of large-bowel perforation in patients with colorectal cancer. Dis Colon Rectum. 1998 Nov; 41(11):1421-6.

[20] Meyer F, Grundmann RT. Hartmann's procedure for perforated diverticulitis and malignant left-sided colorectal obstruction and perforation. Zentralbl Chir. 2011 Feb; 136(1):25-33. Epub 2011 Feb 18.

[21] Min Sang Kim, Seung Woo Lim, Sung Jin Park, Geumhee Gwak, Keun Ho Yang, Byung Noe Bae, Ki Hwan Kim, Sewhan Han, Hong Joo Kim, Young Duck Kim, Hong Yong Kim. Survival Rate and Prognostic Factors in Perforated Colorectal CancerPatients: A Case-Control Study. J Korean Soc Coloproctol: Vol. 26, No. 1, 69-75, 2010.

[22] Khan S, Pawlak SE, Eggenberger JC, Lee CS, Szilagy EJ, Margolin DA. Acute colonic perforation associated with colorectal cancer. Am Surg. 2001 Mar; 67(3):261-4.

[23] Peregudov SI, Sinenchenko GI, Kurygin AA, Pirogov AV. Experience in surgery of diastatic ruptures of the colon. Vestn Khir Im I I Grek. 2008; 167(3):49-53.

[24] Renoux B, Herbault GF, Jean E. Diastatic perforations of the colon of neoplastic origin. Apropos of 15 cases. J Chir (Paris). 1986 Nov; 123(11):644-50.

[25] .Zielinski MD, Merchea A, Heller SF, You YN. Emergency Management of Perforated Colon Cancers: How Aggressive Should We Be? Journal of Gastrointestinal Surgery (Sep 2011).

[26] Iwata T, Konishi K, Yamazaki T, Kitamura K, Katagiri A, Muramoto T, Kubota Y, Yano Y, Kobayashi Y, Yamochi T, Ohike N, Murakami M, Gokan T, Yoshikawa N, Imawari M. Right colon cancer presenting as hemorrhagic shock. World J Gastrointest Pathophysiol. 2011 Feb 15; 2(1):15-8.

[27] Schwartz S et al. Principles of Surgery. Ed I , Teora 2005.pp. 1066-1072

Part 4

Postoperative Follow-Up

5

Surveillance and Characteristics of Recurrence After Curative Resection for Colorectal Cancer

Hirotoshi Kobayashi[1,2] and Kenichi Sugihara[2]
[1]*Center for Minimally Invasive Surgery*
[2]*Department of Surgical Oncology*
Tokyo Medical and Dental University, Tokyo
Japan

1. Introduction

Cancer is the leading cause of death in economically developed countries and the second leading cause of death in developing countries.[1] In developed counties, colorectal cancer is the second leading cause of cancer death in men and the third leading cause of cancer death in women.[2] In developing countries, colorectal cancer is the fifth leading cause of cancer death in men and the sixth in women. Worldwide, colorectal cancer is the fourth leading cause of cancer death in men and the third in women.[2]

The most promising treatment for colorectal cancer is curative surgery. However, some patients recur after curative resection.[3] In order to detect and treat recurrent tumors earlier, a post-operative surveillance after curative resection for colorectal cancer is in clinical use, although an optimal surveillance system for patients with curative resection for colorectal cancer is still uncertain.

In this chapter, we describe some topics concerning surveillance and characteristics of recurrence after curative resection for colorectal cancer as follows:

i. historical review of surveillance
ii. characteristics of recurrence
iii. surveillance tools
iv. recommended surveillance from European Society for Medical Oncology (ESMO), American Society of Clinical Oncology (ASCO), and Japanese Society for Cancer of the Colon and Rectum (JSCCR)

2. Historical review of surveillance after curative resection for colorectal cancer

2.1 Randomized controlled study

The consensus on the optimal surveillance schedule after curative resection for colorectal cancer has not been established. Six randomized controlled trials (RCT) were reported to validate the usefulness of intensive surveillance after curative resection for colorectal cancer (Table 1).[4-9] In all RCTs, there were no differences in recurrence rate between patients with and without intensive follow-up. There was a description of time to recurrence after curative resection for colorectal cancer in three RCTs.[4,5,7] Intensive surveillance led to earlier detection of recurrence in all three RCTs. As for curative resection rates of recurrent tumor, in three RCTs, intensive surveillance led to more frequent curative resection for recurrent tumor.[4,7,9] On the other hand, in two RCTs, there were no differences in resection rates of recurrent tumor.[5,6] Two RCTs disclosed the better survival in the intensive group,[7,9] although the majority of RCTs failed to show a survival benefit of intensive surveillance after curative resection for colorectal cancer.[4-6,8]

2.2 Meta-analysis

Although six RCTs have been conducted, all trials were underpowered or unsatisfactory. Therefore, three meta-analyses using the data of these RCTs evaluated the usefulness of intensive surveillance.[10-12] There was no significant difference in recurrence rate between patients with intensive surveillance and those with non-intensive one. Renehan et al. reported that intensive surveillance led to earlier detection of recurrence after curative resection for colorectal cancer.[12] Jeffery et al. clarified that intensive surveillance led to higher resection rate of recurrent tumor.[11] In all meta-analyses, intensive surveillance improved survival after curative resection for colorectal cancer.

3. Characteristics of recurrence after curative resection for colorectal cancer

The Japanese Society for Cancer of the Colon and Rectum (JSCCR) organized the study group on post-surgical surveillance after curative resection for colorectal cancer in 2003. The data were collected from 14 institutions which were the members of JSCCR. The recurrence rate after curative resection for colorectal cancer was investigated according to the TNM stage and the recurrence site.[3] The data of 5,230 patients who underwent curative resection for colorectal cancer from 1991 to 1996 were collected. Among 5,230 patients, 3,583 had colon cancer and 1,647 had rectal cancer. Among these, 906 patients (17.3%) developed a recurrence during the median surveillance of 6.6 years. The characteristics of patients are shown in Table 2. The recurrence rate was significantly higher in patients with rectal cancer (24.3%) than in those with colon cancer (14.1%, $p<0.0001$).

3.1 Recurrence by TNM stage

The recurrence rate in each stage was 3.7% in stage I, 13.3% in stage II, and 30.8% in stage III, respectively ($p<0.0001$). In each stage, the recurrence rate in patients with rectal cancer was higher than that in patients with colon cancer. The recurrence rates after curative resection for stage I, II, and III colon cancer were 2.7%, 12.1%, and 24.3%, respectively. Those after curative resection for stage I, II, and III rectal cancer were 5.7%, 16.7%, and 43.2%, respectively. The speed of recurrence in patients with stage I cancer was slow and constant (Figure 1a). On the other hand, the recurrence appeared rapidly within 3 years after curative resection for stage II and III colorectal cancer (Figure 1b and 1c). The cumulative appearance rates of recurrence at 3 years for stage I, II, and III were 68.6%, 76.9%, and 87.0%, respectively. Those at 5 years were 96.1%, 92.9%, and 97.8%, respectively. Recurrence after 5 years was rare for all three stages: 0.14% (2/1367), 0.94% (18/1912), and 0.67% (13/1951), respectively.

Author	Year	Number of patients	Study design	Recurrence rate	Time to detection of recurrence	Resection rate of recurrent tumor	Prognosis
Kjeldsen et al. [4]	1997	597	RCT	26% : 26% (NS)	18 months : 27 months ($p<0.01$)	20% : 7% ($p<0.01$)	5-year survival rate 70% : 68% (NS)
Makela et al. [5]	1995	106	RCT	42% : 39% (NS)	10 months : 15 months ($p = 0.002$)	22% : 14% (NS)	5-year survival rate 59% : 54% (NS)
Ohlsson et al. [6]	1995	107	RCT	32% : 33% (NS)	–	29% : 17% (NS)	5-year survival rate 75% : 67% (NS)
Pietra et al. [7]	1998	207	RCT	Local recurrence 25% : 19% (NS)	Local recurrence 10 months : 20 months ($p<0.0003$)	Local recurrence 65% : 10% ($p<0.01$)	5-year survival rate 73% : 58% (NS)
Schoemaker et al. [8]	1998	325	RCT	34%, 41% (NS)	–	–	5-year survival rate 76% : 70% (NS)
Secco et al. [9]	2002	358	RCT	53% : 57%	–	31% : 16% ($p<0.05$)	5-year survival rate in high risk group 50% : 32% ($p<0.05$) 5-year survival rate in low risk group 80% : 60% ($p<0.01$)
Figueredo et al. [10]	2003	1679	Meta-analysis	NS	–	–	Hazard ratio in intensive group 0.80 ($p = 0.0008$)
Jeffery et al. [11]	2002	1342	Meta-analysis	Odds ratio 0.91 (NS)	–	24% : 9%	Hazard ratio in intensive group 0.73 ($p = 0.007$)
Renehan et al. [12]	2002	1342	Meta-analysis	32% : 33% (NS)	8.5 months earlier in intensive group ($p<0.001$)	–	Hazard ratio in intensive group 0.81 ($p = 0.007$)

Table 1. Trials concerning surveillance after curative resection for colorectal cancer

		Patients with relapse (%)	Patients without relapse (%)	Total	P value*
Number of patients		906 (17.3)	4324 (82.7)	5230	
Age		62 ± 11	63 ± 11	63 ± 11	NS**
Gender					
	Male	559 (18.0)	2546 (82.0)	3105	NS***
	Female	347 (16.3)	1778 (83.7)	2125	
Primary tumor site					
	Colon	506 (14.1)	3077 (85.9)	3583	p<0.0001***
	Rectum	400 (24.3)	1247 (75.7)	1647	
TNM stage					
	Stage I	51 (3.7)	1316 (96.3)	1367	
	Stage II	255 (13.3)	1657 (86.7)	1912	p<0.0001***
	Stage III	600 (30.8)	1351 (69.2)	1951	
Median follow-up peric		3.5 ± 2.9	7.1 ± 3.1	6.6 ± 3.1	p<0.0001**

* Characteristics of patients with relapse compared to those without relapse, **Man-Whitney U test, ***chi-square test.

Table 2. Characteristics of patients

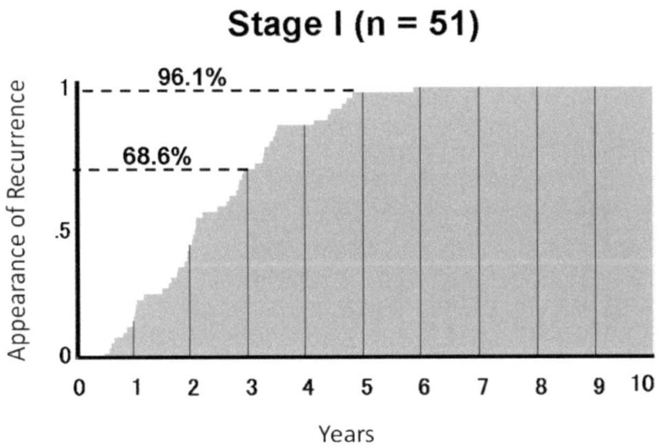

Fig. 1a. The cumulative appearance rate of recurrence after curative resection for stage I (a), stage II (b), and stage III (c) colorectal cancer.

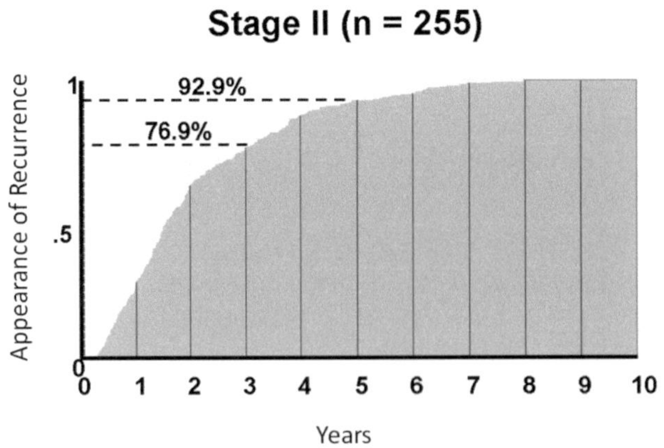

Fig. 1b. The cumulative appearance rate of recurrence after curative resection for stage I (a), stage II (b), and stage III (c) colorectal cancer.

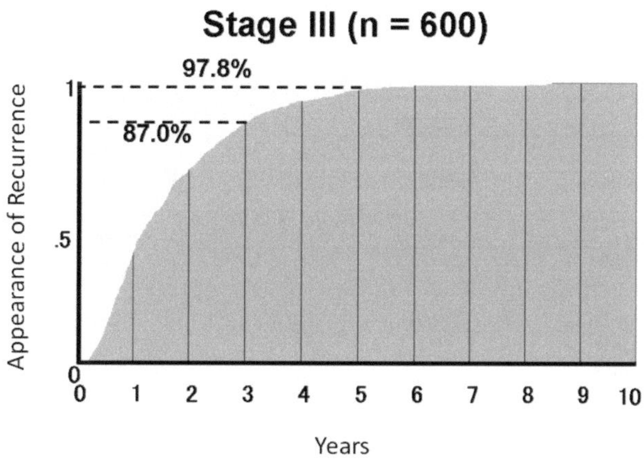

Fig. 1c. The cumulative appearance rate of recurrence after curative resection for stage I (a), stage II (b), and stage III (c) colorectal cancer.

An intensive surveillance program could be adopted in stage II and III patients for the first 3 years and less intensive program for the next 2 years. Patients with stage I colorectal cancer could be followed less intensively.

3.2 First recurrence site

A study using autopsy reported that the most frequent metastatic site from colorectal cancer was the liver followed by the lung.[13] This was consistent with our study (Table 3).[3] The liver was the most frequent recurrent site after curative resection for colon cancer (7.0%). The second was the lung (3.5%). The local recurrence was most frequent after curative resection for rectal cancer (8.8%). The lung and the liver were the second and the third frequent metastatic sites. There was no difference in hepatic recurrence rate between patients with colon cancer and those with rectal cancer, while the pulmonary, local and anastomotic recurrence rates after curative resection for rectal cancer were significantly higher than those for colon cancer. In each recurrent site, approximately 80 to 90% of recurrence developed within 3 years (Figure 2). More than 95% of anastomotic recurrence was found within 3 years after curative resection for colorectal cancer (Figure 2d). In 5 years after curative resection for colorectal cancer, more than 95% of recurrence was found in each recurrent site (Table 4).

In this study, there was no patient with preoperative radiotherapy for rectal cancer. At present, the standard therapy for rectal cancer is total mesorectal excision with preoperative chemoradiotherapy in many countries.[14-18] Six percent of the patients with preoperative combined modality therapy for rectal cancer followed by total mesorectal excision developed a recurrence over 5 years.[19] In their study, of the 67 patients who developed recurrent disease, 4 (6%) had recurrent disease documented greater than 5 years following surgery. Three of these 4 patients had a distant recurrence, and 1 had both a local and distant recurrence. The recurrences were documented 61, 71, 76, and 96 months following curative rectal resection.

Therefore, the surveillance after 5 years might be necessary if patients receive radiotherapy or adjuvant chemotherapy.

		Colon Patients with relapse	(%)	Rectum Patients with relapse	(%)	*P* value*
Number of patients						
		506/3583	(14.1)	400/1647	(24.3)	p<0.0001**
Gender						
	Male	306/2066	(14.8)	253/1039	(24.4)	p<0.0001**
	Female	200/1517	(13.2)	147/608	(24.2)	p<0.0001**
TNM stage						
	Stage I	24/891	(2.7)	27/476	(5.7)	p = 0.0056**
	Stage II	171/1410	(12.1)	84/502	(16.7)	p = 0.0091**
	Stage III	311/1282	(24.3)	289/669	(43.2)	p<0.0001**
First recurrence site						
	Liver	252/3853	(7.0)	121/1647	(7.3)	NS**
	Lung	126/3583	(3.5)	124/1647	(7.5)	p<0.0001**
	Local	64/3583	(1.8)	145/1647	(8.8)	p<0.0001**
	Anastomotic	9/3583	(0.3)	13/1647	(0.8)	p = 0.0052**
	Others	130/3583	(3.6)	69/1647	(4.2)	NS**

* Recurrence rates in patients with colon cancer compared to those with rectal cancer, ** chi-square test, *** Mann-Whitney U test

Table 3. Comparison of recurrence rates between patients with colon cancer and those with rectal cancer

First recurrence site	% recurrence (observed recurrences /5230)	Cumulative appearance rate of recurrence (%) within 3 years	within 4 years	within 5 years
Liver	7.1 (373)	87.9	94.1	98.7
Lung	4.8 (250)	77.7	88.8	94.8
Local	4.0 (209)	81.1	90.3	96.1
Anastomotic	0.4 (22)	95.5	95.5	95.5
Others	3.8 (199)	79.8	91.4	95.5

Table 4. Recurrence rates by the initial recurrence site

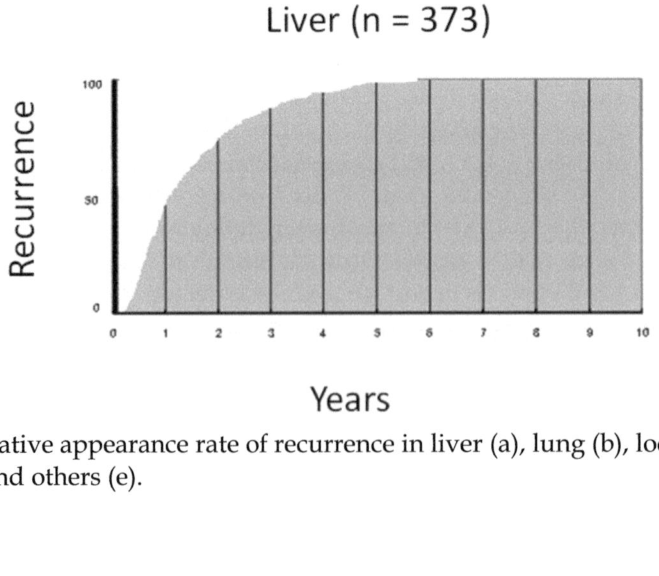

Fig. 2a. The cumulative appearance rate of recurrence in liver (a), lung (b), local (c), anastomosis (d), and others (e).

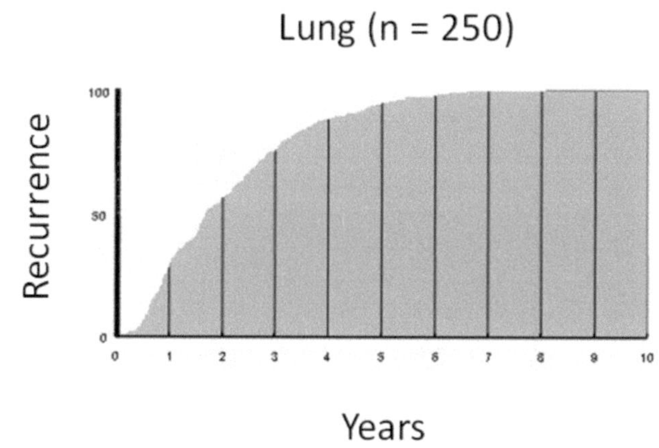

Fig. 2b. The cumulative appearance rate of recurrence in liver (a), lung (b), local (c), anastomosis (d), and others (e).

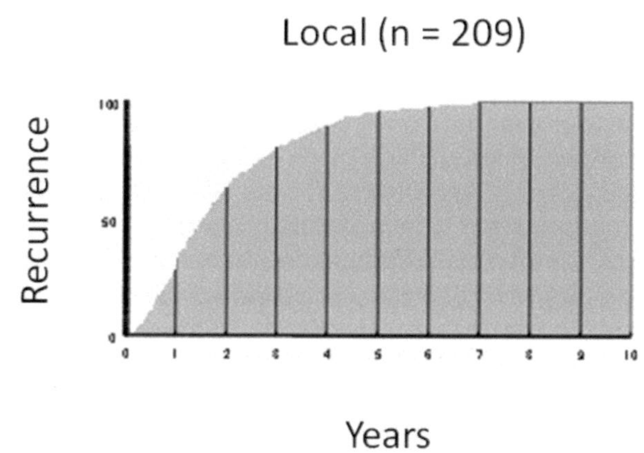

Fig. 2c. The cumulative appearance rate of recurrence in liver (a), lung (b), local (c), anastomosis (d), and others (e).

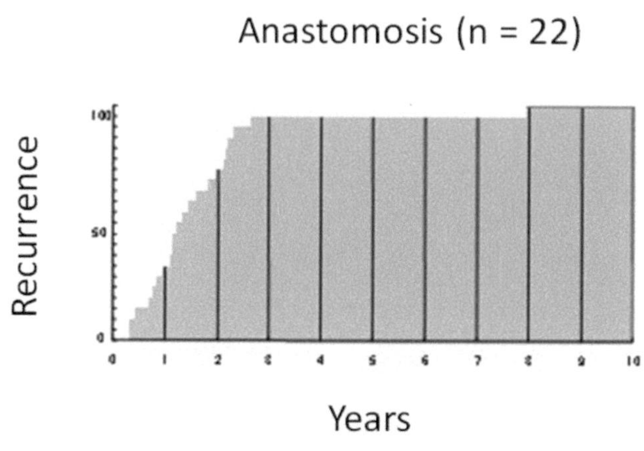

Fig. 2d. The cumulative appearance rate of recurrence in liver (a), lung (b), local (c), anastomosis (d), and others (e).

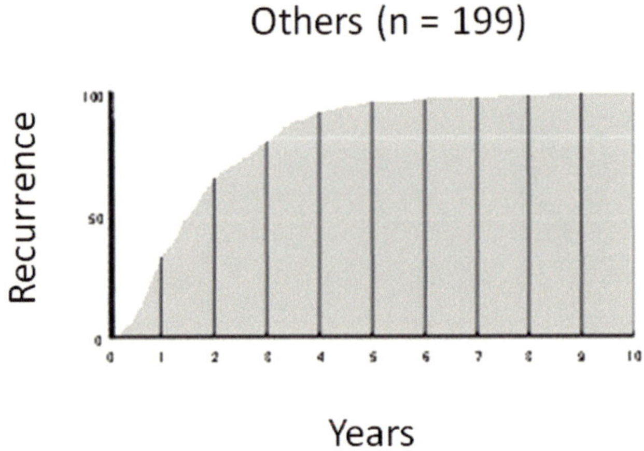

Fig. 2e. The cumulative appearance rate of recurrence in liver (a), lung (b), local (c), anastomosis (d), and others (e).

3.3 Survival

According to the Japanese data, the 5-year overall survival rates in patients with stage I, II, and III colon cancer were 92.8%, 85.5%, and 76.2%, respectively (Figure 3a). Those in patients with stage I, II, and III rectal cancer were 92.2%, 84.6%, and 62.0%, respectively (Figure 3b).[3] These outcomes seem to be better than those of the patients in the Surveillance, Epidemiology, and End Results (SEER) population-based data from 1992 to 2004. According to the SEER data, the 5-year survival rates in patients with stage I, T3N0, and T4N0 colon cancer were 76.3%, 66.7%, and 55.0%, respectively.[20] Those in patients with stage III colon cancer varied from73.7% (T1-2N1a) to 12.9% (T4bN2b).

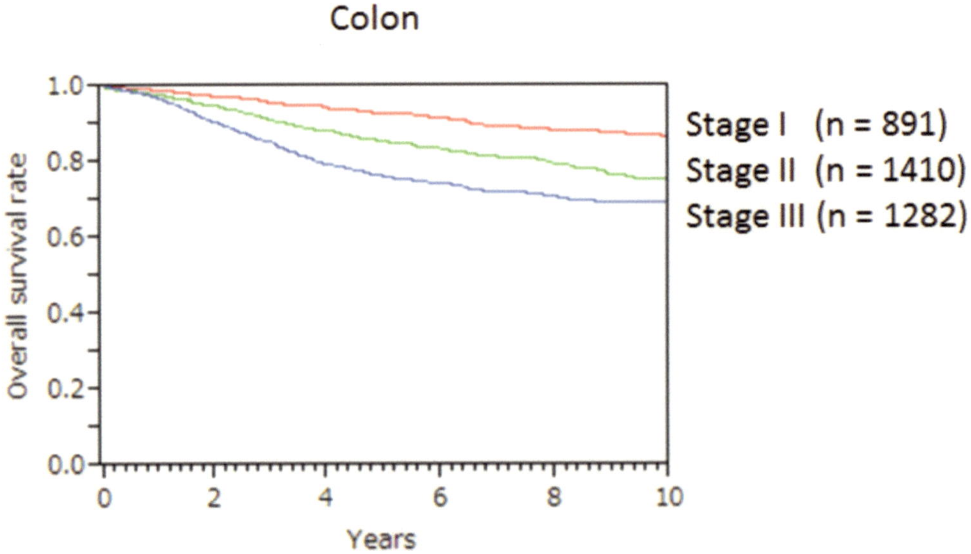

Fig. 3a. The overall survival curve after curative resection for cancer of the colon (a) and rectum (b).

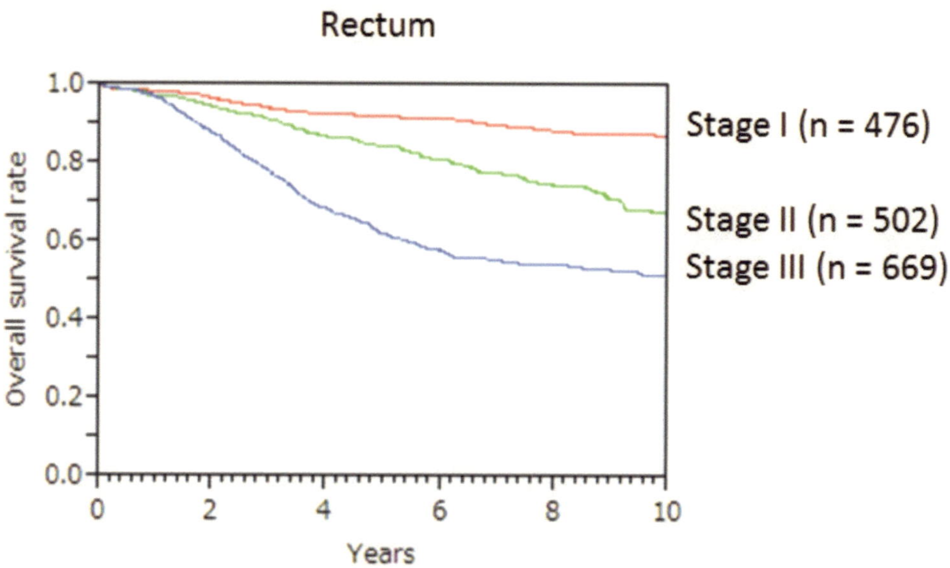

Fig. 3b. The overall survival curve after curative resection for cancer of the colon (a) and rectum (b).

In terms of rectal cancer, the 5-year overall survival rates in Japanese patients with stage I, II, and III rectal cancer were 92.2%, 84.6%, and 62.0%, respectively. According to the SEER data, the 5-year observed survival rates in patients with stage I, T3N0, and T4N0 rectal cancer were 77.6%, 64.0%, and 50.5%, respectively.[21] As for stage III rectal cancer, the 5-year observed survival rates varied from 75.7% (T1N1a) to 12.3% (T4bN2b).

In each stage, the prognosis of the Japanese patients with colorectal cancer was better than that of US patients. One of the possible reasons might be the difference of surveillance system after curative resection for colorectal cancer. The Japanese patients with curative resection for colorectal cancer usually receive more intensive surveillance to detect recurrence than the American patients. Another possible reason might be the difference of surgical technique. The Japanese surgeons usually perform central vascular ligation to dissect regional lymph node. Some European institutions adopt the similar technique called complete mesocolic excision with central ligation. Hohenberger et al. presented an excellent outcome of patients who underwent complete mesocolic excision with central ligation.[22] However, most institutions in the Western countries do not adopt this technique.[23]

3.4 Resection for recurrence

In our study, among the 906 patients with recurrence after curative resection for colorectal cancer, 379 (41.8&) underwent resection for recurrence with curative intent.[3] The prognoses of patients with resection for recurrence were better than those without resection. The 5-year survival rates after initial colorectal surgery in patients with and without resection for hepatic, pulmonary, local, and anastomotic recurrence were 55% and 11% ($p<0.0001$), 68% and 13% ($p<0.0001$), 48% and 22% ($P = 0.0002$), and 53% and 0% ($p = 0.0003$), respectively (Figure 4). The 5-year survival rates after resection for hepatic, pulmonary, local, and anastomotic recurrence were 45%, 48%, 27%, and 33%, respectively.

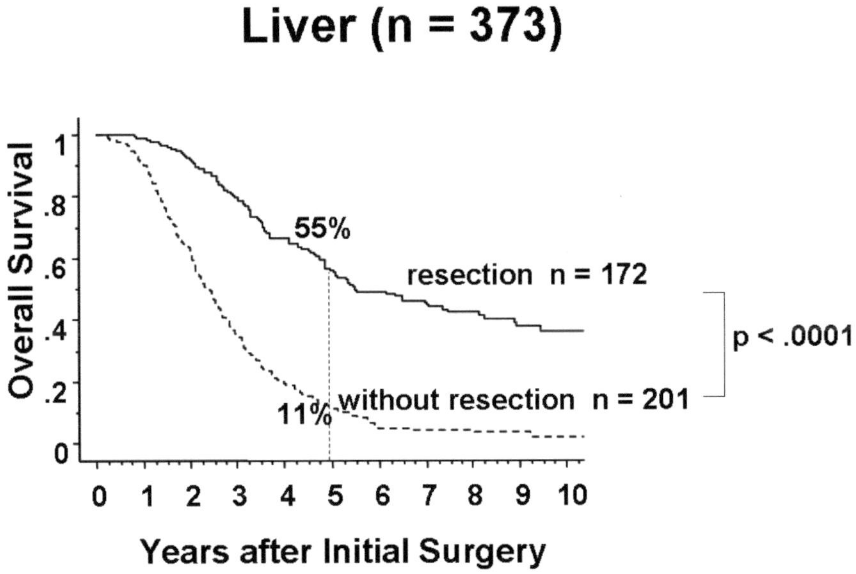

Fig. 4a. The outcomes after initial colorectal surgery in patients with and without resection for recurrence of liver (A), lung (B), local (C), and anastomosis (D).

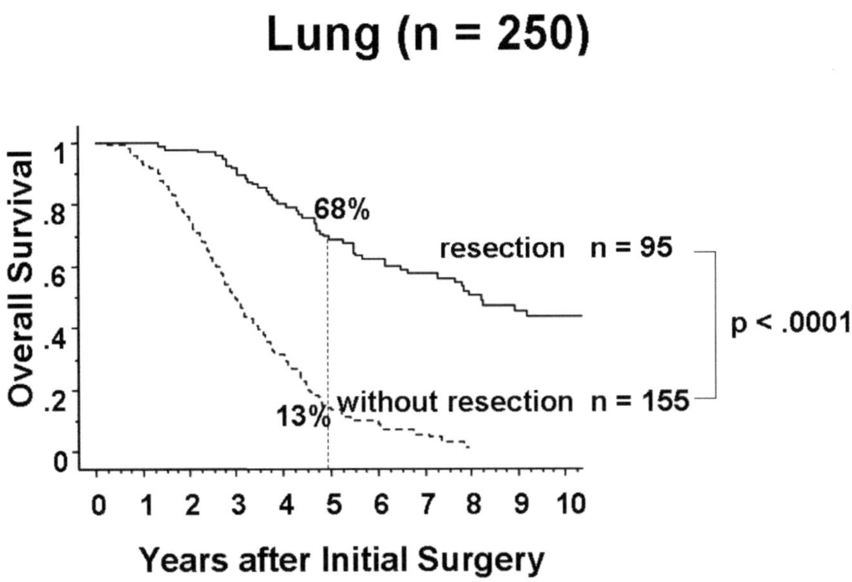

Fig. 4b. The outcomes after initial colorectal surgery in patients with and without resection for recurrence of liver (A), lung (B), local (C), and anastomosis (D).

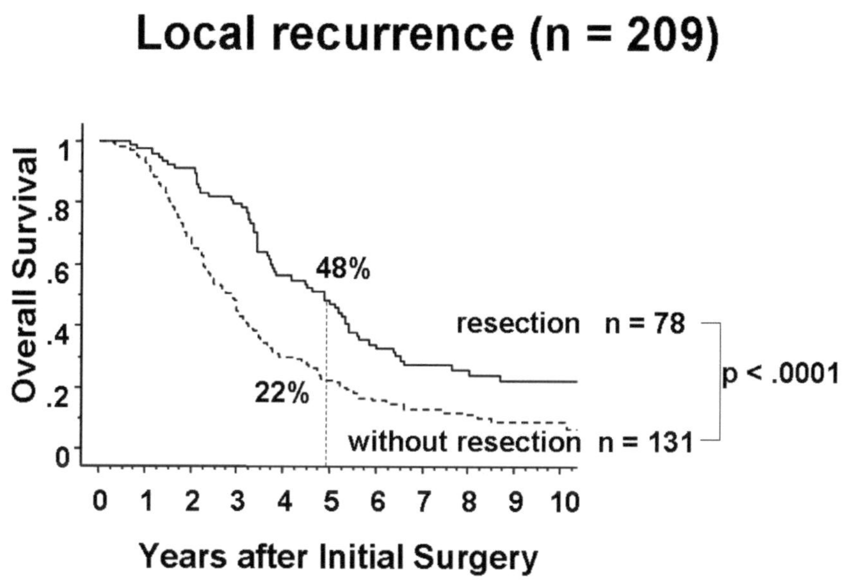

Fig. 4c. The outcomes after initial colorectal surgery in patients with and without resection for recurrence of liver (A), lung (B), local (C), and anastomosis (D).

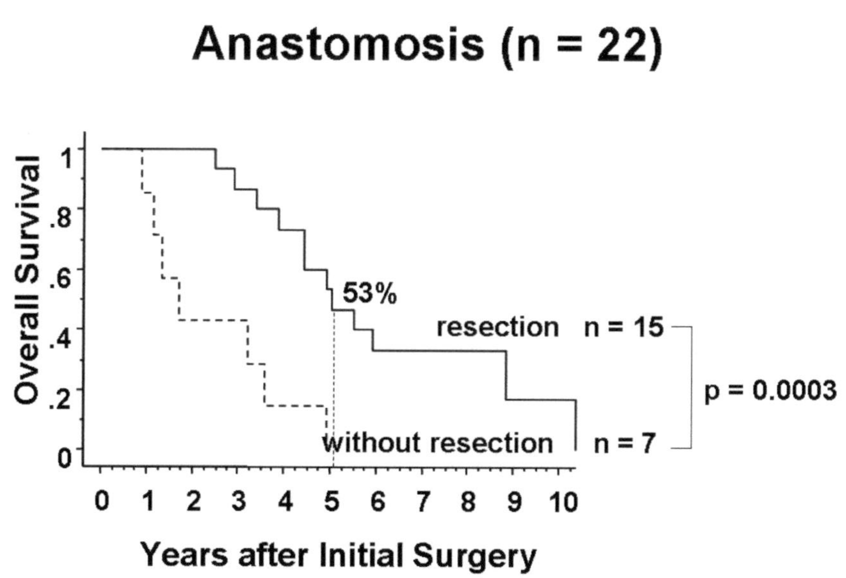

Fig. 4d. The outcomes after initial colorectal surgery in patients with and without resection for recurrence of liver (A), lung (B), local (C), and anastomosis (D).

3.5 Timing of recurrence

Patients were classified into three groups according to the timing of recurrence (TR): TR≤1 year, 1<TR≤3 years, 3 years<TR. The earlier the hepatic, pulmonary, and local recurrence, the poorer the survival after initial colorectal surgery (Figure 5).[24] If patients had resection for recurrence, there was no difference in survival after recurrence according to the timing of recurrence (Figure 6).

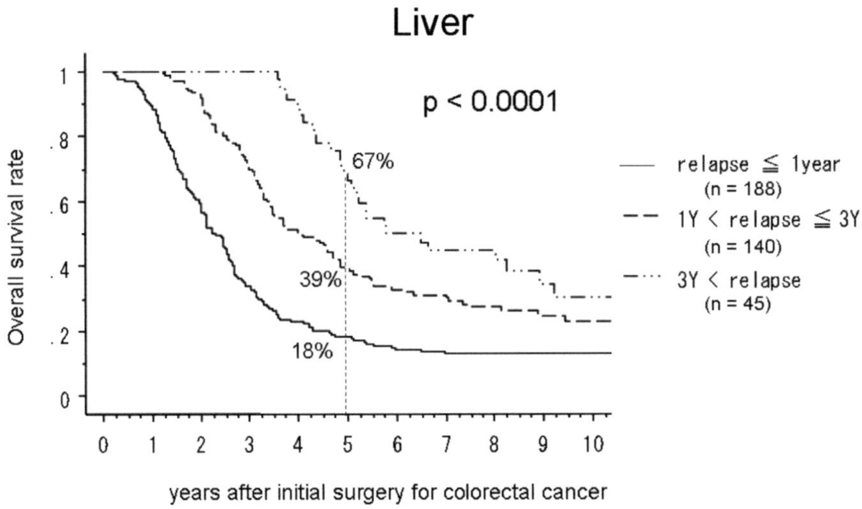

Fig. 5a. The overall survival curve after initial colorectal surgery according to the timing of recurrence. The later recurrence in liver (a), lung (b), and local (c) leads to the better survival.

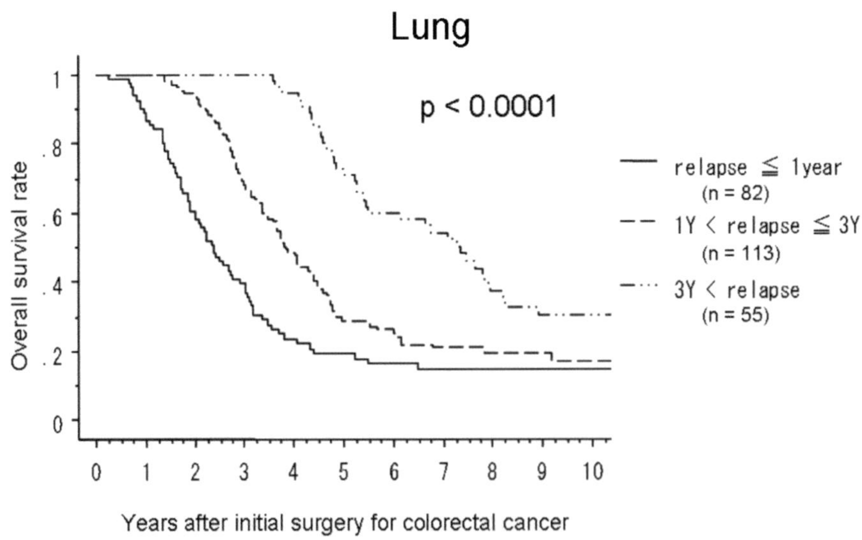

Fig. 5b. The overall survival curve after initial colorectal surgery according to the timing of recurrence. The later recurrence in liver (a), lung (b), and local (c) leads to the better survival.

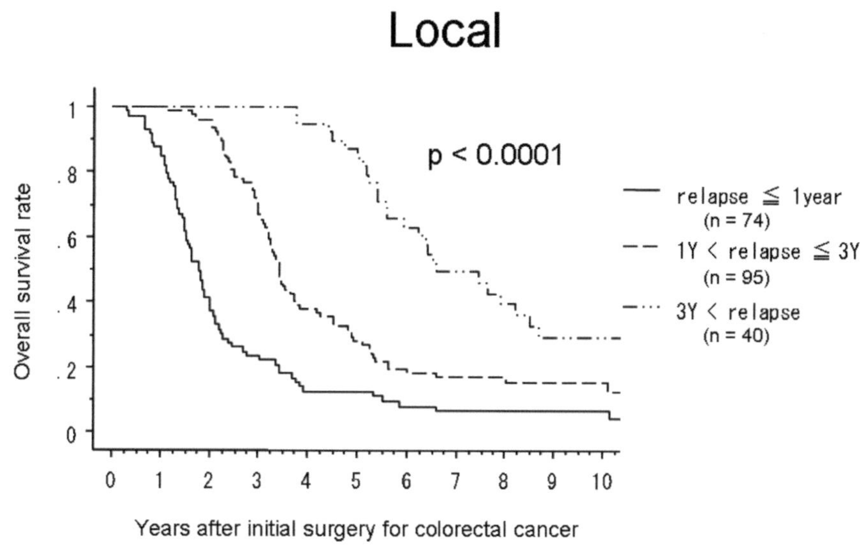

Fig. 5c. The overall survival curve after initial colorectal surgery according to the timing of recurrence. The later recurrence in liver (a), lung (b), and local (c) leads to the better survival.

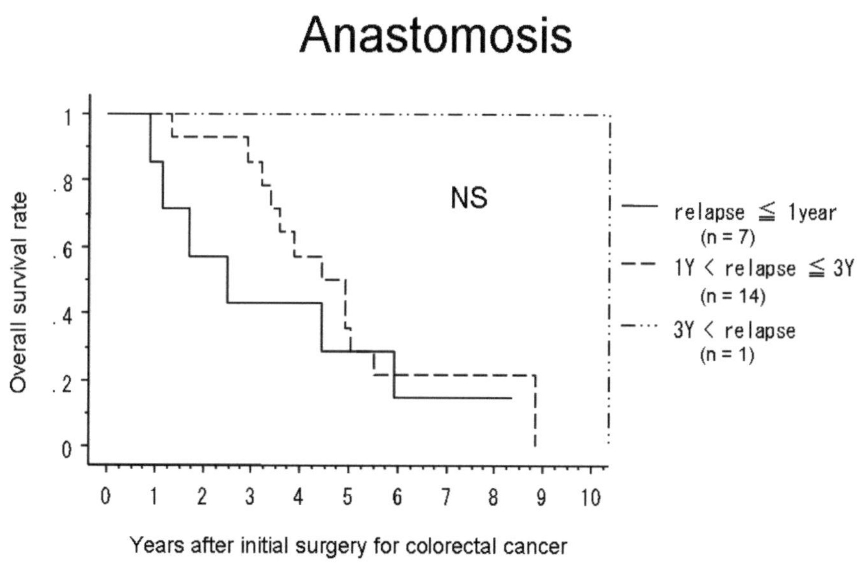

Fig. 5d. The overall survival curve after initial colorectal surgery according to the timing of recurrence. The later recurrence in liver (a), lung (b), and local (c) leads to the better survival.

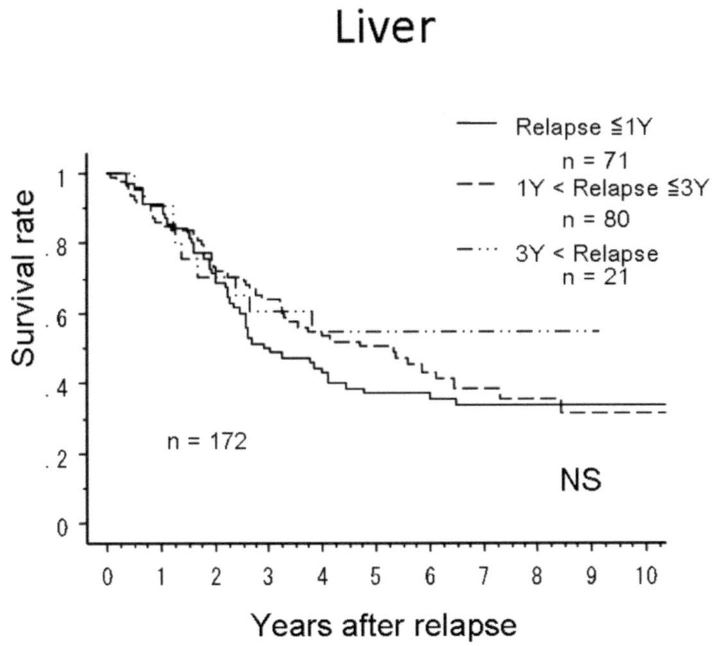

Fig. 6a. If the patients underwent curative resection for recurrence, the outcomes after recurrence were irrespective of the timing of recurrence.

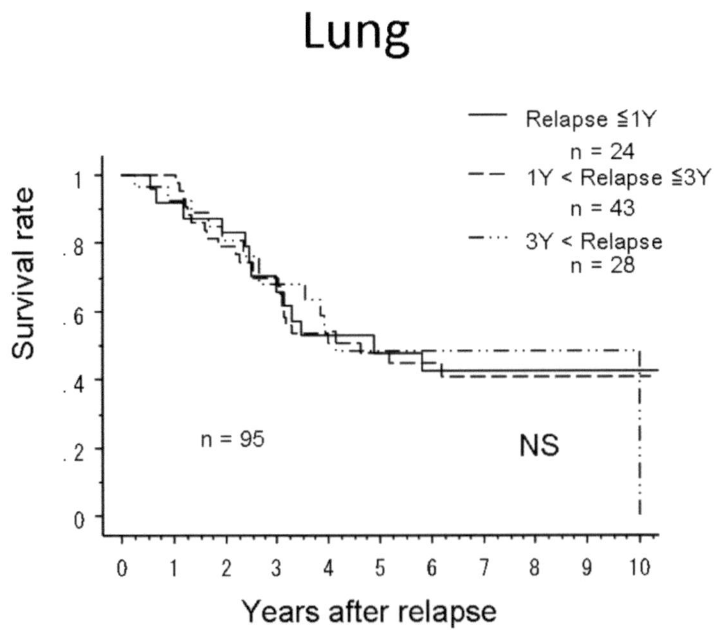

Fig. 6b. If the patients underwent curative resection for recurrence, the outcomes after recurrence were irrespective of the timing of recurrence.

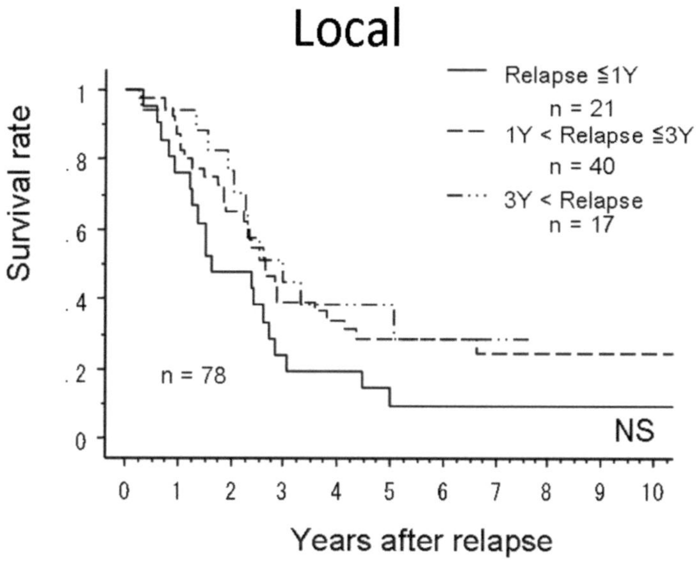

Fig. 6c. If the patients underwent curative resection for recurrence, the outcomes after recurrence were irrespective of the timing of recurrence.

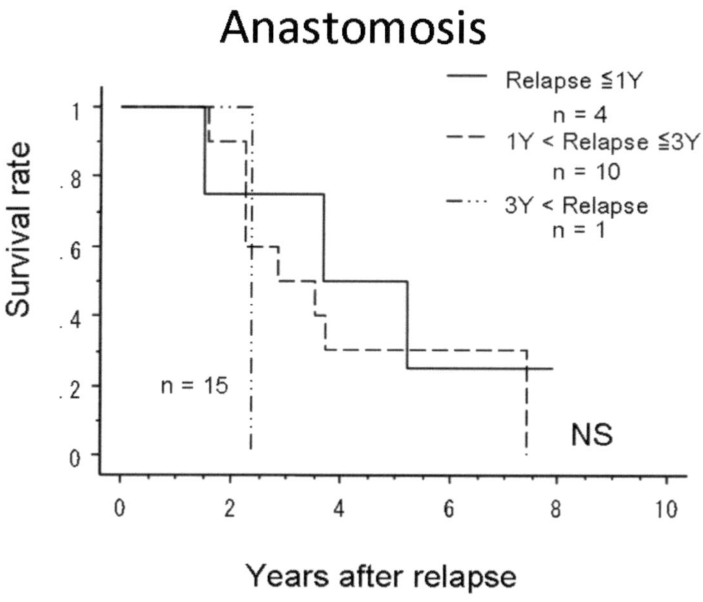

Fig. 6d. If the patients underwent curative resection for recurrence, the outcomes after recurrence were irrespective of the timing of recurrence.

4. Surveillance tools after curative resection for colorectal cancer

In our study, the combination of symptoms, physical examination, and tumor marker detected the majority of recurrence in all sites except for lung (Table 5).[3] In this section, the evidence for usefulness of each surveillance tool is discussed.

First recurrence site	Liver (n = 373)	Lung (n = 250)	Local (n = 209)	Anastomotic (n = 22)	Others (n = 199)
	Rate of FI* (%)	Rate of FI* (%)	Rate of FI* (%)	Rate of FI* (%)	Rate of FI* (%)
A: Symptoms**	3.2	6.8	27.2	13.6	19.6
B: Physical examination	1.6	1.6	20.6	36.4	8.5
C: Tumor marker	46.6	26.4	23.4	18.2	41.7
A + B + C	51.5	34.8	71.3	68.2	69.8
Liver imaging	43.4				
Chest x-ray	1.3	48.4			
CT		10.4	18.2	18.2	18.6
CS***			6.7	9.1	
Others		2.8	2.9		5.5
Unknown	3.8	3.6	1	4.5	6

*FI: First indicator
**Symptoms include anal pain, anal bleeding, abdominal pain, and so on
***CS: Colonoscopy

Table 5. Rate of first indicator for recurrence

4.1 History and physical examination

It is not rare that patients have a symptom at the time of recurrence after curative resection for colorectal cancer. According to the result of RCTs, 16% to 66% of patients had some sort of symptom.[4,5] Therefore, periodical clinical visits seem to be important to detect a recurrence after curative resection for colorectal cancer. On the other hand, Ohlsson et al. reported that it was rare to detect a resectable recurrent tumor only history and physical examination.[6]

4.2 CEA

Carcinoembryonic antigen (CEA) is most widely used as tumor marker for colorectal cancer. The serum CEA level was high in the majority of patients with recurrence after curative resection for colorectal cancer.[25] Especially, 80% of patients with hepatic recurrence from colorectal cancer had higher serum CEA levels.[25] Graham et al. reported that serum CEA measurement was the most useful and economical surveillance tool to detect recurrence after curative resection for colorectal cancer.[26] Therefore, serum CEA test was recommended as a surveillance tool after curative resection for colorectal cancer.[10]

4.3 Chest X-ray

It is controversial to use chest x-ray as a surveillance tool to detect recurrence after curative resection for colorectal cancer. Since chest x-ray can detect resectable pulmonary metastasis with probability of 1%,[26,27] it is not recommended to use chest x-ray as a surveillance tool in many institutions. On the other hand, Ike et al. reported the good outcomes of 42 patients with curative resection for pulmonary recurrence which was detected by the combination of serum CEA test of every 2 months and chest x-ray of every 6 months.[28] The 5-year survival rate after curative resection for pulmonary recurrence was 63.7%.

4.4 CT scans

Howell et al. reported that annual computed tomography (CT) scan could detect 87.5% of liver metastases at an asymptomatic stage,[29] whereas, in total, only 2 cases out of 157 (1.3%) underwent curative resection for liver metastases. An RCT conducted by Schoemaker et al. clarified that abdominal CT scan increased the detection rate of liver metastases, although there was no difference in resection rate between the groups with and without CT scan.[8] On the other hand, the UK group reported the usefulness of serum CEA measurement and CT scan in the surveillance of patients after adjuvant chemotherapy for colorectal cancer.[30] In their study, among 530 patients with stage II and III colorectal cancer, 154 had recurrence after adjuvant chemotherapy. Recurrences were detected by symptoms (n = 65), CEA (n = 45), CT (n = 49), and others (n = 9). The CT-detected group had a better survival compared with the symptomatic group (P =.0046).

Intensive surveillance after curative resection for colorectal cancer was not adopted in Western countries.[31,32] However, since the results of meta-analyses revealed that intensive surveillance after curative resection for colorectal cancer contributed to better outcomes, routine use of CT scans has been recommended.[33,34]

4.5 PET scans

The usefulness of positron-emission tomography (PET) in the detection of recurrence after curative resection for colorectal cancer is uncertain. Sobhani et al. reported a clinical trial that randomly assigned 130 patients with curative resection for colorectal cancer to the conventional surveillance group (periodic serum tumor marker, ultrasound, chest x-ray, and CT scans) and the PET-additional group.[35] The PET scans were performed in 9 and 15 months after surgery. Recurrences were detected after a shorter time (12.1 vs 15.4 months) in the PET group. Moreover, recurrences were more frequently cured by surgery (R0) in the PET group. The usefulness of PET scans in the detection of recurrence after curative resection for colorectal cancer should be clarified in a large-scale study.

4.6 Colonoscopy

Since the anastomotic recurrence rate after colectomy is low, the usefulness of periodical colonoscopy to detect anastomotic recurrence is skeptical.[36] On the other hand, since the anastomotic recurrence rate after resection for rectal cancer is higher than that after resection for colon cancer, several studies reported the adequacy of periodical colonoscopy to detect anastomotic recurrence after surgery.[31,37] At the same time, colonoscopy can find metachronous adenoma and cancer in the colon and rectum. Metachronous lesions develop in 1.5 to 3% of patients in the first 5 years after colorectal surgery.[8,27,38-42] In Japan, the colonoscopy is usually performed one year after colorectal surgery and thereafter every two years. If total colonoscopy cannot be performed preoperatively because of the stenosis, it is recommended that the first colonoscopy should be performed three to six months after colorectal surgery.

5. Recommended surveillance after curative resection for colorectal cancer from ESMO, ASCO, and JSCCR

Both previous and present guidelines for surveillance after curative resection for colorectal cancer from ASCO and ESMO are shown in Table 6.[31,33,34,43] Previously, neither ASCO nor ESMO recommended the intensive surveillance after curative resection for colorectal cancer, because most RCTs failed to show the prognostic significance of intensive surveillance.[4-8] However, since three meta-analyses showed the effectiveness of intensive surveillance, these guidelines changed their attitude toward surveillance after curative resection for colorectal cancer. At present, both societies recommend periodical serum CEA measurement and CT. Periodical colonoscopy to detect metachronous adenoma and cancer is also recommended.

In Japan, JSCCR published the first edition of guidelines for the treatment of colorectal cancer in 2005 and the second edition in 2009. The Japanese institutions adopted more intensive surveillance to detect recurrence after curative resection for colorectal cancer. The recommended surveillance schedule in the Japanese guidelines is shown in the Table 7.

On the other hand, the optimal schedule and modality to detect recurrence after curative resection for colorectal cancer are still uncertain. These issues should be clarified by RCTs in future.

	ASCO		ESMO	
	Previous	Present	Previous	Present
History and physical examination	Every 3 to 6 months for the first 3 years and annually thereafter	Every 3 to 6 months for the first 3 years, every 6 months during years 4 and 5, and subsequently at the discretion of the physician	Every 6 months for 2 years	Every 3 to 6 months for the first 3 years, every 6 months during years 4 and 5
Carcinoembryonic antigen	If resection of liver metastases would be clinically indicated, it is recommended that postoperative serum CEA testing be performed every 2 to 3 months in patients with stage II or III disease for ≥ 2 years after diagnosis.	Every 3 months postoperatively for at least 3 years after diagnosis, if the patient is a candidate for surgery or systemic therapy	Restricted to patients with suspicous symptoms	Every 3–6 months for 3 years and every 6–12 months in years 4 and 5 after surgery if initially elevated
Chest x-ray	May be ordered to diagnose abnormalities prompted by elevated CEA levels or for patients who have symptoms suggestive of a pulmonary metastasis	Not recommended	Restricted to patients with suspicous symptoms	Can be considered every year for 5 years
Chest computed tomography	–	Annually for 3 years after primary therapy for patients who are at higher risk of recurrence and who could be candidates for curative-intent surgery	Restricted to patients with suspicous symptoms	Can be considered for 3 years in patients who are at higher risk for recurrence
Abdominal ultrasonography	Not recommended	–	Annually for 3 years	Every 6 months for 3 years and after 4 and 5 years
Abdominal computed tomography	Not recommended	Annually for 3 years after primary therapy for patients who are at higher risk of recurrence and who could be candidates for curative-intent surgery	Restricted to patients with suspicous symptoms	Can be considered for 3 years in patients who are at higher risk for recurrence
Pelvic computed tomography	Not recommended	For rectal cancer surveillance, especially for patients with several poor prognostic factors, including those who have not been treated with radiation	Not recommended	Restricted to patients with suspicous symptoms
Colonoscopy	Every 3 to 5 years to detect new cancers and polyps	At 3 years after operative treatment, and, if results are normal, every 5 years thereafter; flexible proctosigmoidoscopy every 6 months for 5 years for rectal cancer patients who have not been treated with pelvic radiation	Every 5 years	At 1 year and thereafter every 3–5 years to look for metachronous adenoma and cancers

Table 6. Recommended guidelines from ASCO and ESMO

	Monthes after surgery																			
	3	6	9	12	15	18	21	24	27	30	33	36	39	42	45	48	51	54	57	60
Colon cancer																				
Clinical visit	•	•	•	•	•	•	•	•	•	•	•	•		•		•		•		•
CEA and CA19-9	•	•	•	•	•	•	•	•	•	•	•	•		•		•		•		•
Chest CT		•		•		•		•		•		•		°		•		°		•
Abdominal CT		•		•		•		•		•		•		°		•		°		•
Colonoscopy				•								•								
Rectal cancer																				
Clinical visit	•	•	•	•	•	•	•	•	•	•	•	•		•		•		•		•
CEA and CA19-9	•	•	•	•	•	•	•	•	•	•	•	•		•		•		•		•
Digital examination		•		•		•		•		•		•								
Chest CT		•		•		•		•		•		•		°		•		°		•
Abdominal and pelvic CT		•		•		•		•		•		•		°		•		°		•
Colonoscopy				•				•				•								

•Stage I - Stage III
°Omissible in Stage I and Stage II

Table 7. Surveillance schedule recommended by JSCCR

6. Summary

i. The most frequent site of recurrence after curative resection for colon cancer is the liver. The second is the lung.
ii. The most frequent site of hematogenous recurrence after curative resection for rectal cancer is the lung. The second is the liver.
iii. The recurrence rate in rectal cancer is higher than in colon cancer.
iv. Approximately 80 to 90% of recurrence after curative resection for colorectal cancer developed within 3 years.
v. In any recurrent sites, the prognosis of patients with curative resection for recurrence was better than that of patients without curative resection for recurrence.
vi. The later the recurrence, the better the survival.
vii. If patients undergo curative resection for recurrence, the prognosis after resection for recurrence is irrespective of timing of recurrence.
viii. Although the optimal surveillance tools and schedule are uncertain, the intensive surveillance leads to better survival after curative resection for colorectal cancer compared to the non-intensive one.

7. Reference

[1] World Health Organization. The Global Burden of Disease: 2004 Update. Geneva: World Health Organization; 2008.
[2] Jemal A, Bray F, Center MM, Ferlay J, Ward E, Forman D. Global cancer statistics. CA Cancer J Clin 2011;61:69-90.
[3] Kobayashi H, Mochizuki H, Sugihara K, et al. Characteristics of recurrence and surveillance tools after curative resection for colorectal cancer: a multicenter study. Surgery 2007;141:67-75.
[4] Kjeldsen BJ, Kronborg O, Fenger C, Jorgensen OD. A prospective randomized study of follow-up after radical surgery for colorectal cancer. Br J Surg 1997;84:666-9.
[5] Makela JT, Laitinen SO, Kairaluoma MI. Five-year follow-up after radical surgery for colorectal cancer. Results of a prospective randomized trial. Arch Surg 1995;130:1062-7.
[6] Ohlsson B, Breland U, Ekberg H, Graffner H, Tranberg KG. Follow-up after curative surgery for colorectal carcinoma. Randomized comparison with no follow-up. Dis Colon Rectum 1995;38:619-26.
[7] Pietra N, Sarli L, Costi R, Ouchemi C, Grattarola M, Peracchia A. Role of follow-up in management of local recurrences of colorectal cancer: a prospective, randomized study. Dis Colon Rectum 1998;41:1127-33.
[8] Schoemaker D, Black R, Giles L, Toouli J. Yearly colonoscopy, liver CT, and chest radiography do not influence 5-year survival of colorectal cancer patients. Gastroenterology 1998;114:7-14.
[9] Secco GB, Fardelli R, Gianquinto D, et al. Efficacy and cost of risk-adapted follow-up in patients after colorectal cancer surgery: a prospective, randomized and controlled trial. Eur J Surg Oncol 2002;28:418-23.

[10] Figueredo A, Rumble RB, Maroun J, et al. Follow-up of patients with curatively resected colorectal cancer: a practice guideline. BMC Cancer 2003;3:26.
[11] Jeffery GM, Hickey BE, Hider P. Follow-up strategies for patients treated for non-metastatic colorectal cancer. Cochrane Database Syst Rev 2002:CD002200.
[12] Renehan AG, Egger M, Saunders MP, O'Dwyer ST. Impact on survival of intensive follow up after curative resection for colorectal cancer: systematic review and meta-analysis of randomised trials. BMJ 2002;324:813.
[13] Weiss L, Grundmann E, Torhorst J, et al. Haematogenous metastatic patterns in colonic carcinoma: an analysis of 1541 necropsies. J Pathol 1986;150:195-203.
[14] Randomised trial of surgery alone versus surgery followed by radiotherapy for mobile cancer of the rectum. Medical Research Council Rectal Cancer Working Party. Lancet 1996;348:1610-4.
[15] Improved survival with preoperative radiotherapy in resectable rectal cancer. Swedish Rectal Cancer Trial. N Engl J Med 1997;336:980-7.
[16] Kapiteijn E, Marijnen CA, Nagtegaal ID, et al. Preoperative radiotherapy combined with total mesorectal excision for resectable rectal cancer. N Engl J Med 2001;345:638-46.
[17] Adjuvant radiotherapy for rectal cancer: a systematic overview of 8,507 patients from 22 randomised trials. Lancet 2001;358:1291-304.
[18] Camma C, Giunta M, Fiorica F, Pagliaro L, Craxi A, Cottone M. Preoperative radiotherapy for resectable rectal cancer: A meta-analysis. Jama 2000;284:1008-15.
[19] Guillem JG, Chessin DB, Cohen AM, et al. Long-term oncologic outcome following preoperative combined modality therapy and total mesorectal excision of locally advanced rectal cancer. Ann Surg 2005;241:829-36; discussion 36-8.
[20] Gunderson LL, Jessup JM, Sargent DJ, Greene FL, Stewart AK. Revised TN categorization for colon cancer based on national survival outcomes data. J Clin Oncol 2010;28:264-71.
[21] Gunderson LL, Jessup JM, Sargent DJ, Greene FL, Stewart A. Revised tumor and node categorization for rectal cancer based on surveillance, epidemiology, and end results and rectal pooled analysis outcomes. J Clin Oncol 2010;28:256-63.
[22] Hohenberger W, Weber K, Matzel K, Papadopoulos T, Merkel S. Standardized surgery for colonic cancer: complete mesocolic excision and central ligation--technical notes and outcome. Colorectal Dis 2009;11:354-64; discussion 64-5.
[23] West NP, Hohenberger W, Weber K, Perrakis A, Finan PJ, Quirke P. Complete mesocolic excision with central vascular ligation produces an oncologically superior specimen compared with standard surgery for carcinoma of the colon. J Clin Oncol 2010;28:272-8.
[24] Kobayashi H, Mochizuki H, Morita T, et al. Timing of relapse and outcome after curative resection for colorectal cancer: a Japanese multicenter study. Dig Surg 2009;26:249-55.
[25] McCall JL, Black RB, Rich CA, et al. The value of serum carcinoembryonic antigen in predicting recurrent disease following curative resection of colorectal cancer. Dis Colon Rectum 1994;37:875-81.

[26] Graham RA, Wang S, Catalano PJ, Haller DG. Postsurgical surveillance of colon cancer: preliminary cost analysis of physician examination, carcinoembryonic antigen testing, chest x-ray, and colonoscopy. Ann Surg 1998;228:59-63.
[27] Safi F, Link KH, Beger HG. Is follow-up of colorectal cancer patients worthwhile? Dis Colon Rectum 1993;36:636-43; discussion 43-4.
[28] Ike H, Shimada H, Ohki S, Togo S, Yamaguchi S, Ichikawa Y. Results of aggressive resection of lung metastases from colorectal carcinoma detected by intensive follow-up. Dis Colon Rectum 2002;45:468-73; discussion 73-5.
[29] Howell JD, Wotherspoon H, Leen E, Cooke TC, McArdle CS. Evaluation of a follow-up programme after curative resection for colorectal cancer. Br J Cancer 1999;79:308-10.
[30] Chau I, Allen MJ, Cunningham D, et al. The value of routine serum carcino-embryonic antigen measurement and computed tomography in the surveillance of patients after adjuvant chemotherapy for colorectal cancer. J Clin Oncol 2004;22:1420-9.
[31] Desch CE, Benson AB, 3rd, Smith TJ, et al. Recommended colorectal cancer surveillance guidelines by the American Society of Clinical Oncology. J Clin Oncol 1999;17:1312.
[32] Tveit KM. ESMO Minimum Clinical Recommendations for diagnosis, treatment and follow-up of rectal cancer. Ann Oncol 2003;14:1006-7.
[33] Desch CE, Benson AB, 3rd, Somerfield MR, et al. Colorectal cancer surveillance: 2005 update of an American Society of Clinical Oncology practice guideline. J Clin Oncol 2005;23:8512-9.
[34] Van Cutsem EJ, Oliveira J. Colon cancer: ESMO clinical recommendations for diagnosis, adjuvant treatment and follow-up. Ann Oncol 2008;19 Suppl 2:ii29-30.
[35] Sobhani I, Tiret E, Lebtahi R, et al. Early detection of recurrence by 18FDG-PET in the follow-up of patients with colorectal cancer. Br J Cancer 2008;98:875-80.
[36] Anthony T, Fleming JB, Bieligk SC, et al. Postoperative colorectal cancer surveillance. J Am Coll Surg 2000;190:737-49.
[37] Fleischer DE, Goldberg SB, Browning TH, et al. Detection and surveillance of colorectal cancer. JAMA 1989;261:580-5.
[38] Barillari P, Ramacciato G, Manetti G, Bovino A, Sammartino P, Stipa V. Surveillance of colorectal cancer: effectiveness of early detection of intraluminal recurrences on prognosis and survival of patients treated for cure. Diseases of the colon and rectum 1996;39:388-93.
[39] Bruinvels DJ, Stiggelbout AM, Kievit J, van Houwelingen HC, Habbema JD, van de Velde CJ. Follow-up of patients with colorectal cancer. A meta-analysis. Ann Surg 1994;219:174-82.
[40] Green RJ, Metlay JP, Propert K, et al. Surveillance for second primary colorectal cancer after adjuvant chemotherapy: an analysis of Intergroup 0089. Ann Intern Med 2002;136:261-9.
[41] Juhl G, Larson GM, Mullins R, Bond S, Polk HC, Jr. Six-year results of annual colonoscopy after resection of colorectal cancer. World J Surg 1990;14:255-60; discussion 60-1.

[42] Ringland CL, Arkenau HT, O'Connell DL, Ward RL. Second primary colorectal cancers (SPCRCs): experiences from a large Australian Cancer Registry. Annals of oncology : official journal of the European Society for Medical Oncology/ESMO 2010;21:92-7.

[43] ESMO Minimum Clinical Recommendations for diagnosis, adjuvant treatment and follow-up of colon cancer. Ann Oncol 2001;12:1053-4.

6

Difficult Infected Wound After Colorectal Surgery

Prem Rathore
The Townsville Hospital, James Cook University, Queensland Australia

1. Introduction

Surgical site infection (SSI) is a well known and commonly encountered scenario following major colorectal resection and has been documented as being a potentially morbid and costly complication.

Surgical wounds in normal, healthy individuals heal through an orderly sequence of physiologic events that include inflammation, epithelialisation, fibroplasia, and maturation. Mechanical failure or failure of wound healing at the surgical site can lead to disruption of the closure leading to seroma, hematoma, wound dehiscence or hernia. Other complications include surgical site infection and nerve injury.

For this reason, of late, emphasis has been placed on more efficient management of these patients including early recognition, and prompt treatment with a view to improve patient outcomes which are measured both in terms of postoperative morbidity, prolonged hospital stay and by extension an increased demand on finite hospital resources[1].

However, there has been wide discrepancy in the reported incidence of incisional SSI following colorectal surgery, ranging from 3 to 30%[(1)]. Additionally, there has been no clear consensus on the risk factors contributing to SSI following colorectal surgery, which has limited the data's value to surgeons involved in quality improvement programs hoping to address specific variables that could reduce this risk.

In this era of managed care organizations where patients expect short hospital stay and one-stage resections are becoming more frequent, peri operative assessment of risk factors for wound infection should be intensified for the patient.

Surgical site infections (SSI) are the third most common hospital-acquired infection and account for 14% to 16% of all such infections. However, in surgical patients, SSI is the leading cause of hospital-acquired infection[2,3]. Similar incidence of SSI has been documented by various studies in patients after colorectal surgery.

The National Nosocomial Infection Surveillance system surveys all colorectal surgeries together, without differentiating the type of colorectal surgery performed. The outcome of their survey showed rectal surgery may have a higher risk for SSI, and identifying risk factors that are more specific to this procedure would be a better indicator to predict the possibility of SSI.

Several reports have described the substantial cost of these infections in terms of attributable mortality,[3] increased morbidity measured as increased postoperative hospital length of stay, and increased hospital costs.

2. Risk factors

Various studies have identified multiple risk factors and other associations which have a direct bearing on the incidence of these infections.

a. **Type of surgery:** Timing of the surgical procedure does not significantly predispose or preclude wound infections as it occurs in patients who have undergone both emergency surgery as well as those that had an elective procedure.
b. **Patient related risk factors for surgical site infection**[4] *(Table 1)*: This group of risk factors have a significant impact on the incidence of surgical site infection. Included in this group are pre-existing conditions like diabetes and cardiovascular disease. Patients nutritional status - both malnutrition and obesity and life style habits like smoking can cause significant impact on post-operative wound. Prior medical history of surgery, irradiation or cancer also adversely effect wound healing.

1.	Diabetes
2.	Obesity
3.	Immunosuppression
4.	Cardiovascular disease
5.	Smoking
6.	Cancer
7.	Previous surgery
8.	Malnutrition and
9.	Prior irradiation

Table 1. Patient Related Risk Factors for Surgical Site Infection [4]

c. **Technique related risk factors for surgical site infection**[4] *(Table 2)*: Various surgical related factors affect wound healing differently. This includes both pre surgical patient preparation and post operative care. Intra operative procedures including the surgical techniques like excessive use of electrocautery, poor haemostasis and tissue trauma can adversely affect wound healing as can the length of the surgery. Insertion and duration of intra abdominal drains remains a controversial point.

1.	Use of electrocautery	9.	Operating room ventilation
2.	Closure of subcutaneous tissue	10.	Inadequate sterilisation of instruments
3.	Duration of surgical scrub		
4.	Skin antisepsis	11.	Foreign material in the surgical site
5.	Preoperative shaving	12.	Surgical drains
6.	Preoperative skin prep	13.	Poor haemostasis
7.	Duration of operation	14.	Failure to obliterate dead space
8.	Antimicrobial prophylaxis	15.	Tissue trauma

Table 2. Technique Related Risk Factors For Surgical Site Infection [4]

d. **Factors associated with increased risk of fascial disruption**[5] *(Table 3)*: Multiple factors can increase the changes of loss of integrity of the fascia and largely relate to patient factors including patients' premorbid and associated medical conditions as does patient demographics.

1. Age > 65 years 2. Emergency surgery 3. Anemia: hemotocrit <30 percent 4. Obesity: body mass index >30 kg/m^2 5. Ascites 6. Diabetes mellitus 7. Pulmonary disease, COPD, chronic cough	8. Shock 9. Poor nutrition: albumin <3.5 g/dL 10. Infection 11. Immunosuppressive therapy, glucocorticoids, antineoplastic agents 12. Jaundice 13. Male gender

Table 3. Factors associated with increased risk of fascial disruption

3. Classification of abdominal wound infection

Surgical wound infection can be classified into different types based on various criteria[6].

a. Based on the depth and the site of the surgical wound infection, the three types are:
   1. **Superficial incisional surgical site infection**: Involves skin and subcutaneous fat (Image 1).
   2. **Deep incisional surgical site infection**: Involves rectus sheath and preperitoneal space (Image 2).
   3. **Organ / space surgical site infection**: Involves intraperitoneal compartment and intra abdominal organs (Image 3).

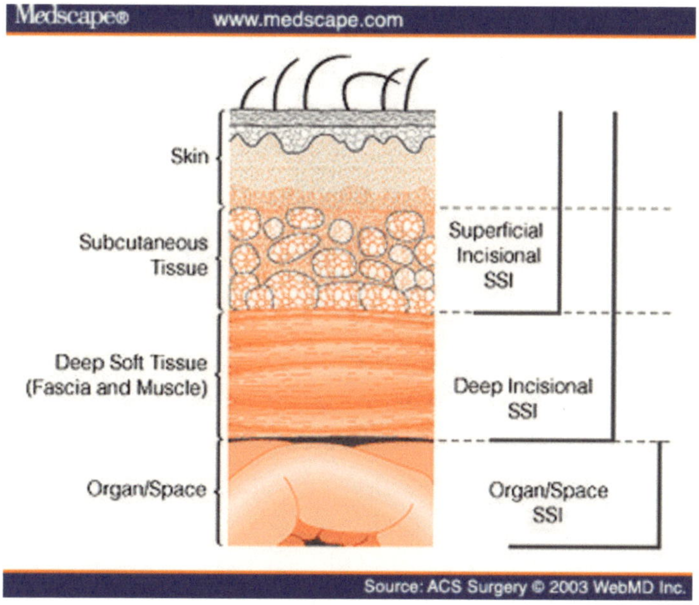

Fig. 1.

b. Based on the type of wound they are classified as:
   1. **Clean**
   2. **Clean contaminated**
   3. **Contaminated**
   4. **Dirty**

Studies have shown an association between the type of wound and the incidence of surgical site infection (Table 4):

Classification	Examples	Incidence of SSI (%)
Clean	Elective surgery without violation of the gut or infected spaces	< 2
Clean contaminated	Elective bowel surgery (prepared bowel, mechanical and antibiotic)	5-15
Contaminated	Emergent bowel surgery (unprepared bowel, minor spillage), drainage of infected spaces	15-30
Dirty	Grossly contaminated traumatic wounds, significant intestinal spillage, grossly infected and devitalized tissue (necrotizing infection)	>30

Table 4. Wound Classification and Risk for Surgical Site Infection

4. Clinical manifestation and diagnosis

As with infection anywhere, surgical site infections present with localized erythema, induration, warmth, and pain at the incision site. Purulent wound drainage and separation of the wound may occur.

Some patients will have systemic evidence of their infection such as fever and leukocytosis.

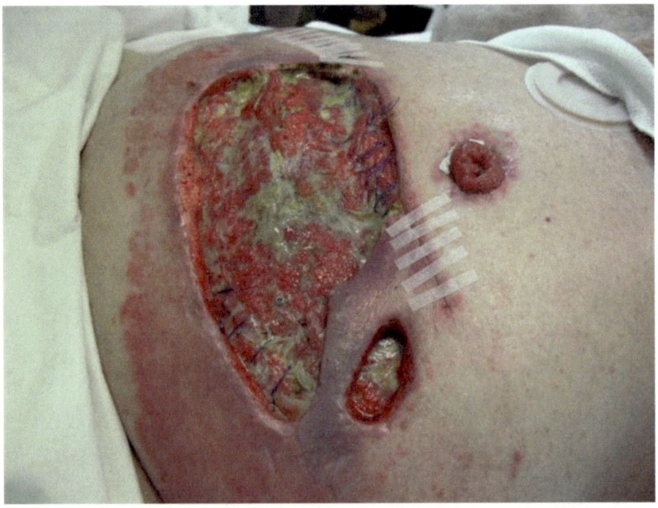

Image 1. Superficial incisional surgical site infection showing skin and subcutaneous fat involvement.

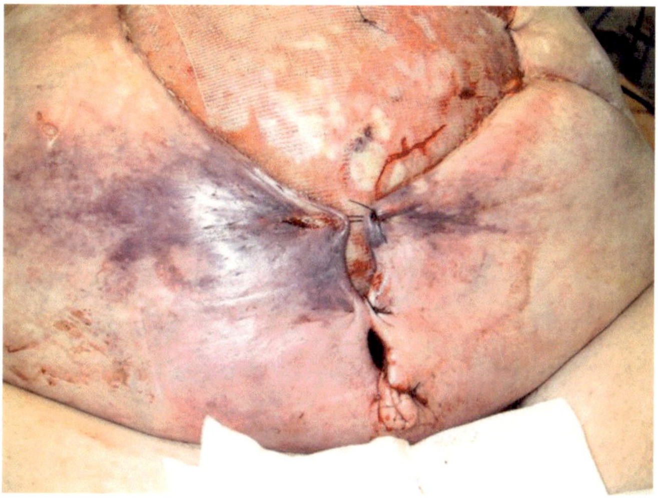

Image 2. Deep incisional surgical site infection involving rectus sheath and preperitoneal space.

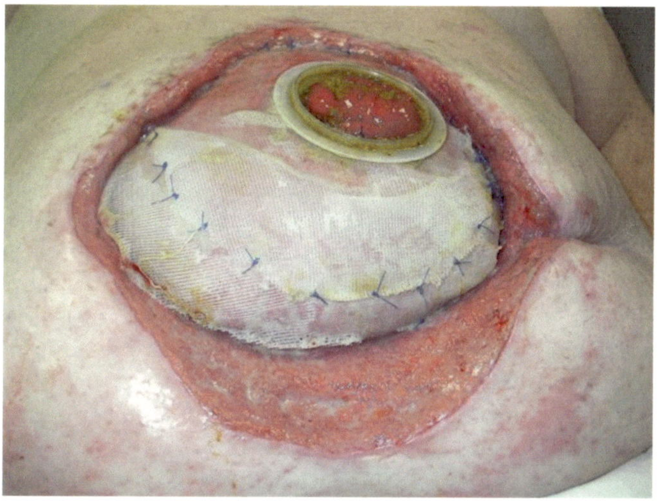

Image 3. Organ surgical site infection shown as an open abdomen with Involvement of the peritoneal cavity and omentum managed by mesh placement.

Diagnosis of surgical site infection is largely clinical.

Role of imaging is limited to those patients in whom there is a clinical suspicion of deep space infections or collections. Of the imaging modalities, Computed Tomography is the preferred modality for assessment.

Ultrasound may have a limited role in assessing deep space infections but can evaluate collections related to superficial wounds, particularly, if the clinical evaluation is difficult or inconclusive.

5. Complication of SSI

In addition to the complications related directly to the wound, patients with SSI can have other complications based on their pre surgical risk factors and co morbidities that can adversely affect their long term outcome and prolong their convalescence.

These complications have been well documented and researched and include long hospital stay, increasing morbidity, SIRS - Sepsis - MOF and even death.

5.1 Management

Recent studies have shown the strong influence of the various risk factors that results in an increase in the incidence of surgical site infection. Thus, there has been a shift in the approach to the management of these patients with emphasis being placed on prophylaxis.

5.1.1 Prophylaxis

- Adequately identifying and correcting the various systemic co-morbidities thus optimising the pre-operative status and reducing the pre-operative risk for SSI.
- This has shown to be as important as post-operative and intra-operative care. It includes ensuring adequate control of diabetes and assessment and correction of cardiovascular problems pre-operatively.
- Studies have shown that cessation of smoking at least a week prior to surgery reduces the risk of SSI.
- Both reduction of weight in obese patients and improvement of nutrition in cachectic patients have shown to favourably improve surgical outcome.
- Optimising surgical techniques at various levels starting with adequate patient preparation for surgery which include antibacterial shower on the day of surgery, shaving of the site on table.
- Adequate antimicrobial prophylaxis which is continued intra operatively at 4 hourly intervals.
- Mass closure of the abdominal wound incorporating all layers of the rectus sheath taking wide tissue bites of more than 1cm and with short stitch interval (less than 1cm) using suture length to wound length ratio of 4 to 1.
- Reducing tissue trauma during surgery by gentle dissection of tissue, cautious use of electrocautery and saline wash-out of the wound has shown a lower incidence of SSI. Reducing operative time and appropriate use of intrabdominal drains also reduces the risk.
- **Best practices for preventing surgical site infections [7]:**

Evidence category IA - Well designed studies

1. Cancel elective surgery if the patient has an infection at or remote from the surgical site
2. Achieve maximal subcutaneous concentration of peri operative antibiotics
3. Maintain prophylactic antibiotics for only a few hours after closing incisions
4. If it is necessary to remove hair, use clippers, not shaving, immediately before operation

Evidence category IB - Good evidence and expert consensus

1. Control glucose levels in diabetic patients and avoid peri operative hyperglycemia

2. Encourage patients who use tobacco products to quit using or to abstain for 30 days prior to surgery
3. Have the patient shower or bathe with an antiseptic agent on at least the night before surgery
4. Follow strict standards for sterilizing instruments, disinfecting operating room, and air circulation
5. Do not routinely use vancomycin for prophylaxis if other agents are appropriate
6. Do not use UV radiation in the operating room for infection prophylaxis
7. Surgical staff who have draining skin lesions are excluded from duty
8. Surgical staff should wear sterile clothing and gloves
9. Surgical team hand hygiene to include keeping fingernails short, scrubbing with antiseptic to elbows for 2-5 min, using sterile towels
10. Use appropriate topical microbicides during surgery
11. Use proper surgical technique
12. Apply sterile dressing to incision for 24-48 hours postoperatively and wash hands before contact with surgical site
13. Perform hospital surveillance for surgical site infection

5.1.2 Definitive management

Definitive management of SSI depends on the type of infection.

5.1.2.1 Superficial incisional surgical site infection

Infected wounds are opened, explored, drained, irrigated, débrided and dressed open.

If fascial disruption is suspected, drainage should be performed in the operating room.

The severity of the infection determines the need for antibiotic therapy. Once the infection has cleared and granulation tissue is apparent, the wound can be closed secondarily.

5.1.2.2 Deep incisional surgical site infection

Fascial dehiscence:

Fascial disruption is due to abdominal wall tension overcoming tissue or suture strength, or knot security as a result of infection or collection. It can occur either early or late in the postoperative period and can involve a portion of the incision (i.e, partial dehiscence) or the entire incision (i.e, complete fascial dehiscence).

The incidence of fascial disruption ranges from 0.4 to 3.5 % depending upon the type of surgery performed. Despite improved perioperative care and stronger suture materials, the incidence and morbidity of fascial dehiscence is largely unchanged.

When fascial disruption is suspected, wound exploration should be performed in the operating room. Complete fascial dehiscence is associated with a mortality rate of 10% and is a surgical emergency. At the bedside, a moist dressing is placed over the wound and a binder placed around the patient's abdomen to prevent evisceration on the way to the operating room.

Once opened, the wound is thoroughly debrided. Treatment options include either using VAC dressing or mass closure. Mass closure done with continuous or retention non-absorbable sutures is an option only if the intra-abdominal pressure and tissue oedema intraoperatively is not high. In such cases VAC dressing is the preferred treatment.

Prevention

Meta-analyses related to abdominal fascial closure suggest an optimal technique for closure of abdominal surgical wounds includes[8,9]:

- Use of a simple running technique
- Use of #1 or #2 delayed absorbable monofilament suture
- Use of mass closure to incorporate all layers of the abdominal wall (except skin)
- Taking wide tissue bites (≥1 cm)
- Use of a short stitch interval (≤1 cm)
- Use of a suture length to wound length ratio of 4 to 1
- Use of non-strangulating tension on the suture.

5.1.2.3 Organ/Space surgical site infection

One of the critical decisions in the surgical treatment of patients with severe peritonitis is whether to use an open-abdomen or a closed-abdomen technique.

Closed abdomen technique

The goal of the closed-abdomen technique is to provide definitive surgical treatment at the initial operation which saves the patient from repetitive trauma of anaesthesia and surgery.

Opting for this technique should be judicious in an unstable patient.

Open abdomen technique

VAC dressing and temporary closure with sponge or mesh are types of open abdomen techniques which are valuable tools for the management of patients with acidosis, hypothermia and coagulopathy. This is a very resource-intensive decision.

The goal of the open-abdomen technique is to provide easy, direct access to the affected area. Source control is achieved through repeated reoperations or through open packing of the abdomen. This technique may be well suited for initial damage control in extensive peritonitis.

The open-abdomen technique should also be considered in patients who are at high risk for the development of abdominal compartment syndrome (eg, patients with intestinal distension, extensive abdominal wall and intra-abdominal organ edema), because attempts to perform primary fascial closure under significant tension in these circumstances are associated with an increased incidence of multiple organ failure (eg, renal, respiratory), necrotizing abdominal wall infections, anastomotic leak, entero-cutaneous fistula and mortality.

Temporary closure of the abdomen to prevent herniation and contamination can be achieved by using various materials (Table 5):

1. Self-adhesive impermeable membrane dressings using sponge and opsite. Though it is in inexpensive and easy to apply, the major disadvantage is difficulty in maintaining wound seal. In addition, there is loss of large volumes of extracellular fluid.
2. Mesh like Vicryl and Dexon made of absorbable material can be directly applied over bowel, but the drawbacks are loss of strength in the presence of infection and higher incidence of ventral hernia development.

Closure Technique	Description	Advantages	Disadvantages
Self-adhesive impermeable membranes	Abdominal dressing with gauze and coverage of the entire wound with impermeable membrane with and without placement of drains between the layers	Inexpensive Easy application	Difficult to maintain seal Potentially large volume losses Fistula formation
Vicryl or Dexon mesh	Suturing of the mesh to the fascial edges; different options for dressing	Can be applied directly over bowel Allows for drainage of peritoneal fluid	Rapid loss of tensile strength (in the setting of infection) Potentially large volume losses Higher incidence of later ventral hernia development No reopen-and-close option Fistula formation
Polypropylene mesh	Suturing of the mesh to the fascial edges; different options for dressing	Good tensile strength Allows for drainage of peritoneal fluid	Risk of intestinal erosion when applied directly over bowel Potentially large volume losses High risk of mesh infection Fistula formation
GORE-TEX mesh	Suturing of the mesh to the fascial edges; different options for dressing	Good tensile strength Reopen and close option	Potential fluid accumulation underneath the mesh Limited tissue integration and granulation tissue formation over the mesh Risk of mesh infection Fistula formation
Human acellular dermis	Suturing of the mesh to the fascial edges	Good tensile strength	Expensive Needs 10 minutes of rehydration
Vacuum-assisted closure device	Sponges applied over mesh and attached to controlled, low-level suction	Controlled drainage of secretions Accelerated granulation tissue formation Wound debridement Can remain in place for longer than 48 hours	Cost Risk of intestinal erosion when applied directly over bowel Fistula formation
Wittmann patch	Suturing of artificial burr (ie, Velcro) to fascia, staged abdom-inal closure by application of controlled tension	Good tensile strength Allows for easy re exploration and eventual primary fascial closure	Fistula formation

Table 5. Temporary closure materials.

3. Non absorbable mesh like GORE-TEX and polypropylene can be used for closure with or without zipper. These materials have good tensile strength and provide additional option of repeated surgeries. The disadvantage, however, is mesh erosion into the bowel wall forming fistula and subsequent high risk of mesh infection.

4. Vacuum assisted closure device has the advantage of controlled drainage of secretions. It can also be left in situ for more than 48 hours which is adequate time for the patient to recover from systemic conditions like coagulopathy or metabolic acidosis (Damage control surgery). Increased cost is a major limiting factor against widespread use.

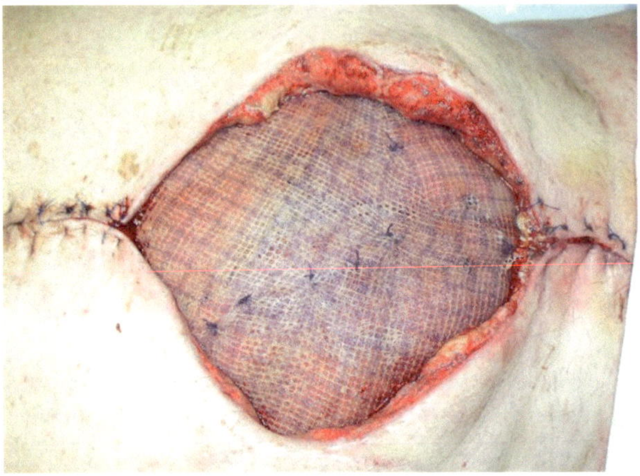

Image 4. Open abdomen technique (mesh)

6. Emerging new techniques for management of open abdomen

6.1 Abdominal vacuum-assisted closure (V.A.C.) systems[10,11]

The V.A.C.® Abdominal Dressing System is a specialty dressing indicated for temporary bridging of the open abdomen where primary closure is not possible and/or repeat abdominal entries are necessary.

The V.A.C. Abdominal Dressing System can be used to assist in the management of an open abdomen due to Abdominal Compartment Syndrome, trauma requiring damage control or staged abdominal repair, and other complex abdominal pathologies.

V.A.C systems are intended to create an environment that promotes wound healing by secondary or delayed primary intention by preparing the wound for closure, reducing edema, promoting granulation tissue formation and perfusion and by removing exudative and infectious material.

These systems are indicated for patients with open abdomen and dehisced wounds, partial-thickness burns, chromic ulcers (such as diabetic, pressure or venous insufficiency).

The V.A.C. GranuFoam™ Silver Dressing is an effective barrier to bacterial penetration and may help reduce infection in the above wound types.

Placement of V.A.C systems directly in contact with exposed blood vessels, anastomotic sites, organs, or nerves is contraindicated. V.A.C. Therapy is also contraindicated for patients with malignancy in the wound, untreated osteomyelitis, non-enteric and unexplored fistulas and necrotic tissue with eschar present.

However, after debridement of necrotic tissue and complete removal of eschar, V.A.C. Therapy may be used.

Following initiation of V.A.C Therapy, the wound can be re evaluated after 72 hours. This can either be done at the bed-side under sedation or under anaesthesia in the theatre. If the wound continues to be infected or dirty, the V.A.C system is reapplied. On the other hand, if the wound is clean, then the decision to proceed to secondary closure of the abdomen can be made.

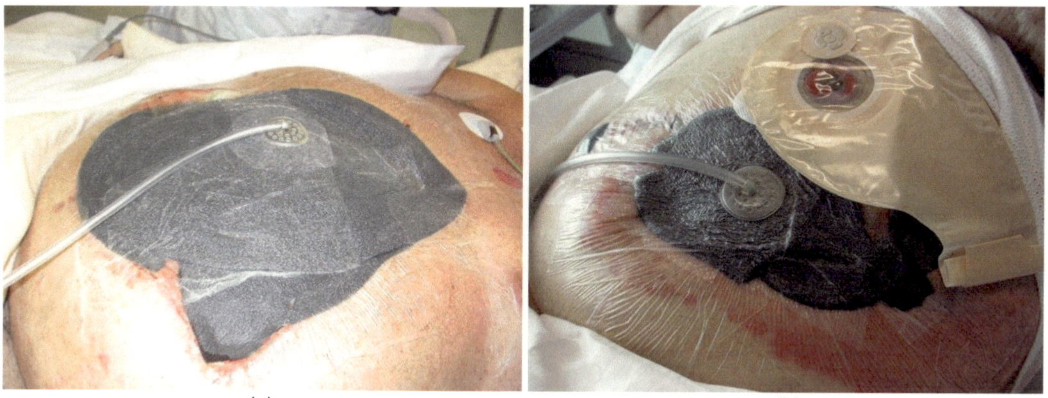

(a) (b)

Image 5. a,b: V.A.C Therapy for open abdomen

6.2 Mist therapy [12]

MIST Therapy® is a painless, noncontact, low frequency ultrasound delivered through a saline mist to the wound bed.These gentle sound waves stimulate the cells within and below the wound bed to promote healing.

The result of these gentle sound waves pushing against the tissue include:

- Cell stimulation
- Reduced inflammation
- Reduced bacteria and bio burden
- Increased blood flow

7. Summary

Surgical site infection (SSI) is a well known and commonly encountered scenario following major colorectal resection and has been documented as being a potentially morbid and costly complication.

Risk factors for surgical site infection include: smoking, diabetes, malnutrition, cancer, obesity, immunosuppression, cardiovascular disease and prior incision or irradiation at the surgical site. Meticulous surgical technique that avoids excessive tissue injury and ischemia while providing adequate hemostasis are important for preventing infection.

Surgeons can modify rates of infection with preventive measures that include antibiotic prophylaxis, proper skin preparation and maintenance of sterile conditions intra operatively. Proper surgical technique with gentle tissue handling and a secure closure that does not cause tissue ischemia are also important.

Infected wounds are opened, explored, drained, irrigated, débrided and dressed open. If fascial disruption is suspected, drainage should be performed in the operating room. The severity of the infection determines the need for antibiotic therapy. Once the infection has cleared and granulation tissue is apparent, the wound can be closed secondarily.

Fascial disruption is due to abdominal wall tension overcoming tissue or suture strength, or knot security. It can occur early or late in the postoperative period. With early fascial dehiscence, the skin closure may be intact depending upon the method of closure (ie, staples, sutures); the patient, nevertheless, is at risk for evisceration. Early postoperative fascial dehiscence is a surgical emergency. The late complication of fascial disruption is incisional hernia which can lead to bowel obstruction, ischemia and even death.

Management of the deep incisional surgical site and organ/space surgical site infection includes open abdomen technique using various types of dressings and mesh. Occasionally, single stage closure of the abdomen is used.

Of late, V.A.C dressings are the preferred choice for open abdomen management. However, the most recent development is the MIST therapy using low frequency ultrasound.

8. References

[1] Robert L. Smith, MD, Jamie K. Bohl, MD, Shannon T. McElearney, MD, Charles M. Friel, MD, Margaret M. Barclay, RN, ACNP-C, Robert G. Sawyer, MD, and Eugene F. Foley, MD :Wound Infection After Elective Colorectal Resection. *Annals of Surgery* v.239(5);May 2004.

[2] Coppa GF, Eng K, Gouge TH, et al. Parenteral and oral antibiotics in elective colon and rectal surgery. A prospective, randomized trial. *Am J Surg*. 1983;145:62- 65.

[3] Tang R, Chen HH, Wang YL, et al. Risk factors for surgical site infection after elective resection of the colon and rectum: a single-center prospective study of 2,809 consecutive patients. *Annals of Surgery* 2001;234:181–9.

[4] SHEA, APIC, CDC, SIS. Consensus paper on the surveillance of surgical wound infections. *Infect Control Hosp Epidemiol* 1992; 13:599.

[5] Cruse PJ. Surgical wound infection. *In: Infectious Diseases*, Wonsiewicz MJ (Ed), WB Saunders Co, Philadelphia 1992. p.7583:599.

[6] Mangram AJ, Horan TC, Pearson ML, etal. Guideline for prevention of surgical site infection. *In: Infection Control and Hospital Epidemiology*, CDC 1999; 20:24

[7] Adapted from the Centers for Disease Control Guidelines for Prevention of Surgical Site Infection (www.cdc.gov/ncidod/dhqp/gl_surgicalsite.html).

[8] Ceydeli A, Rucinski J, Wise L. Finding the best abdominal closure: an evidence-based review of the literature. *Curr Surg* 2005; 62:220

[9] Finding the best abdominal closure: an evidence-based review of the literature.AU Ceydeli A, Rucinski J, Wise LSO, Curr Surg. 2005;62(2):220.

[10] Vacuum-Assisted Closure of Postoperative Abdominal Wounds: A Prospective Study. Sriram Subramonia, Sarah Pankhurst, Brian J. Rowlands and Dileep N. Lobo, *World Journal of Surgery*, Volume 33, Number 5, 931-937, DOI: 10.1007/s00268-009-9947-z.

[11] Alvarez AA, Maxwell GL, Rodriguez GC, *Gynecol Oncol.* 2001Mar;80(3):413-6.

[12] Howell M. Case study 000090-000307-000928 www.celleration.com